Current Problems in Dermatology

Vol. 38

Series Editor

P. Itin Basel

Management of Psoriasis

Volume Editor

Nikhil Yawalkar Bern

30 figures, 30 in color, and 11 tables, 2009

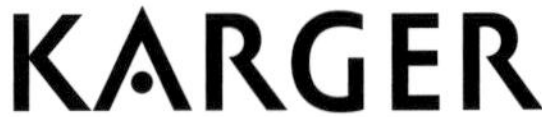

Basel · Freiburg · Paris · London · New York · Bangalore · Bangkok · Shanghai · Singapore · Tokyo · Sydney

Current Problems in Dermatology

Nikhil Yawalkar
University Hospital Bern
Department of Dermatology
Inselspital
CH–3010 Bern/Switzerland

Library of Congress Cataloging-in-Publication Data

Management of psoriasis / volume editor, Nikhil Yawalkar.
p. ; cm. -- (Current problems in dermatology ; v. 38)
Includes bibliographical references and index.
ISBN 978-3-8055-9151-5 (hard cover : alk. paper)
1. Psoriasis. I. Yawalkar, Nikhil. II. Series: Current problems in dermatology ; v. 38.
[DNLM: 1. Psoriasis--therapy. W1 CU804L v.38 2009 / WR 205 M266 2009]
RL321.M36 2009
616.5′26--dc22

2009017067

Bibliographic Indices. This publication is listed in bibliographic services, including Current Contents® and Index Medicus.

www.karger.com
Printed in Switzerland on acid-free and non-aging paper (ISO 9706) by Reinhardt Druck, Basel
ISSN 1421-5721
ISBN 978-3-8055-9151-5
e-ISBN 978-3-8055-9152-2

Contents

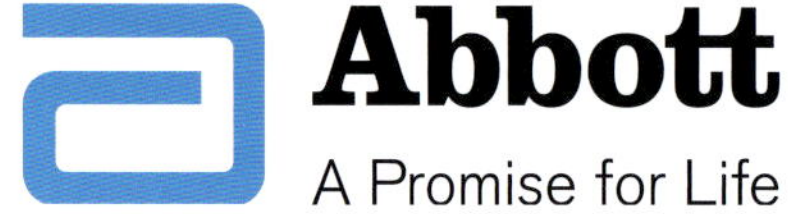

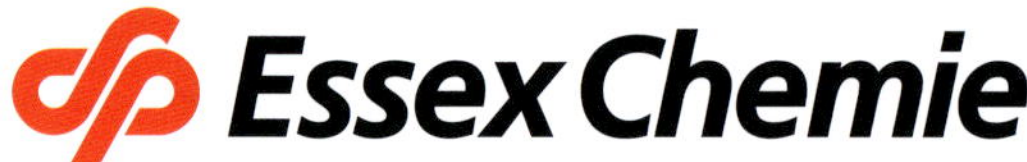

Wyeth

This book has been printed with the financial support from Abbott, Essex AG and Wyeth.

Preface

Psoriasis is a chronic, currently incurable, inflammatory skin disease with considerable clinical heterogeneity, which affects approximately 2% of the population. Since skin diseases like psoriasis are not usually life-threatening, their negative impact on individuals is often underestimated by society and even by health care professionals. However, the comparison of psoriasis with other chronic debilitating medical and psychiatric conditions confirms that psoriasis produces an immense detriment in quality of life. Furthermore, a proportion of psoriasis patients are still frustrated and dissatisfied with the overall treatment and management of their disease. Psoriasis is increasingly recognized as being associated with a higher rate of comorbidities, like depression, psoriatic arthritis, Crohn's disease and, particularly in severe psoriasis, metabolic syndrome and cardiovascular diseases. The reasons for the latter associations still remain to be fully elucidated, and may involve genetic and lifestyle factors (nicotine or alcohol abuse, high-fat foods, lack of regular physical exercise, stress) and possibly the degree of psoriatic skin inflammation. The presence of comorbidities, like metabolic syndrome and cardiovascular diseases, may profoundly influence the treatment options, e.g. by contraindications to antipsoriatic medications (acitretin, cyclosporine). Moreover, the association between psoriasis and the above-mentioned comorbidities make an interdisciplinary treatment approach together with the general practitioner, psychiatrists, rheumatologists, cardiologists and/or diabetologists of increasing importance.

In recent years, great advances have been made in the understanding of the pathogenesis of psoriasis. This has lead to novel systemic immunomodulatory therapies (biologicals), which are characterized by more specific targeting of defined molecules in the pathological pathways involved in psoriasis. Such biologicals may achieve acute and long-term disease control, with improvements in the quality of life of a significant amount of patients with moderate-to-severe psoriasis. Although the efficacy of many of these agents is unquestionable, the safety of long-term treatment needs to be firmly established in the coming years. This is an tremendously exciting and demanding time for psoriasis patients and dermatologists, who practically every year are confronted with the approval of novel therapies and an immense amount of information on psoriasis. However, many well-established and trusted treatments also exist, which may achieve disease control in numerous patients. It is fundamental that dermatologists are well informed about both conventional and novel psoriasis treatments, and use them correctly to minimize toxicity and maximize efficacy and adherence to therapy. Thus, therapy of psoriasis nowadays can be quite challenging, and includes knowledge about effects and side effects of various drugs, as well as consideration of many factors including age, severity, phenotype, localization, comorbidities, response and contraindications to therapies, trigger factors (like infections and concomitant drugs) and, last but not least, the patient's perception, quality of life and social factors.

This textbook has been written by renowned experts on psoriasis and comprehensively describes clinical features, comorbidities and treatment modalities, including topical therapies, different phototherapeutic options, and both conventional and novel systemic psoriasis treatments. It also includes chapters on the management of childhood psoriasis and psoriasis treatment in difficult locations, like the scalp, face, flexures, palm/soles and nails. I have invited experts with years of practical experience in dealing with psoriatic patients to summarize the relevant aspects of daily psoriasis management, and have also particularly encouraged them to include their personal viewpoints and treatment strategies. It is hoped that the information in this book will be useful for trainee and practising dermatologists, as well as non-dermatologists, and help to improve the management and quality of life of all of our patients with mild or moderate-to-severe psoriasis.

I would like to thank the international panel of distinguished authors for their time and effort, as well as the staff of Karger for their support with this project. We are also very grateful to Abbott, Essex and Wyeth for their financial support. Finally, I would like to dedicate this book to my family for their wonderful support and love.

Nikhil Yawalkar
Bern

Yawalkar N (ed): Management of Psoriasis.
Curr Probl Dermatol. Basel, Karger, 2009, vol 38, pp 1–20

Clinical Spectrum and Severity of Psoriasis

Matthew Meier · Pranav B. Sheth

Department of Dermatology, University of Cincinnati College of Medicine, Cincinnati, Ohio, USA

Abstract

Psoriasis is a chronic inflammatory skin disease. Associated comorbidities or risks may include psoriatic arthritis, obesity, depression, smoking, diabetes, hyperlipidemia, an increased risk of cardiovascular disease with myocardial infarction, or an increased risk of lymphoma. The clinical presentation of psoriasis can range from the more common red scaling elevated plaques on the elbows, knees, or scalp to the less common superficial pustules scattered on the palms or soles, or in rare cases widespread pustules on the body. More specifically, the clinical spectrum of psoriasis includes the plaque, guttate, small plaque, inverse, erythrodermic, and pustular variants. The determinants of the clinical severity of psoriasis, the risk of comorbidities, and the quality of life of a psoriatic patient are influenced by multiple factors. At the minimum, these include variations in the quality and type of psoriasis, the quantity of skin involved, and the distribution of skin lesions (including special areas such as the scalp, nails, face, intertriginous regions, and palmoplantar surfaces). Objective measures used to quantify the severity of psoriasis, including the body surface area involved, Physician's Global Assessment, Psoriasis Area and Severity Index, and quality of life measures, are all assessments that can be useful in guiding approaches to management and therapeutics. In this paper, we review the clinical spectrum of psoriasis, the differential diagnoses, measures and determinants of severity, and the recommendations on when to refer a patient to a specialist in psoriasis. We also briefly review the comorbidities, and note the importance of referring the psoriatic patient to the internist/general practitioner for evaluation and management for these comorbidities.

Psoriasis is a chronic inflammatory disorder of the skin that can affect a person at any age. It can present in various patterns and forms. The most common morphologic presentation of psoriasis is that of the plaque type, with the second form being the pustular type. Its course is variable and unpredictable. It may be episodic with short or long periods of reported complete clearance, or be unrelenting and persistent with waxing and waning of activity influenced by identifiable or unidentifiable triggers and alleviators. Initially it may be indolent and virtually unrecognizable as 'psoriasis' by the patient or physician, only to present itself in a more classic presentation during times of emotional, physical, or medical stress.

Throughout history, psoriasis has been understood and misunderstood as a disease solely of the skin. Its consequences on the social, psychological, physical, and spiritual fabric of the individual and those close to him/her have been increasingly recognized. However, by the end of the 20th century, the psoriasis model had evolved to become a disorder of the skin and joints. Accepted as the consequence of an immune system gone awry, psoriasis has become a model of a skin disease with 'systemic inflammation'. Much work is now being done to understand the association of comorbidities with psoriasis and their impact on the patient and society.

With the advances in technology and medical research, the current pathogenetic model for psoriatic disease includes a combination of genetic predisposition, immunologic dysfunction, and keratinocyte factors that lead to the formation of psoriasis. Along with these, the roles of the peripheral and central nervous systems, vascular system, adaptive and innate immune systems, environmental factors, and infectious agents contribute to the formation of psoriasis. In this paper, we will review the clinical spectrum, the differential diagnosis, and the severity of psoriasis as they relate to quality of life, therapeutic options, and signs that indicate when further evaluation by a dermatologist or a specialist in psoriatic disease is warranted.

Epidemiology

It is estimated that approximately 2% of the US population is affected by psoriasis. Similar prevalence values have been obtained in Europe, with the exception of slightly higher values seen in Norway and the Faeroe Islands. Racial differences do exist. In a recent US population-based survey, the prevalence in Caucasians was estimated to be 2.5%, while in African-Americans this was 1.3%. Males and females are affected equally. Psoriasis can present at any age, but most commonly presents in bimodal peaks between the ages of 15 and 30, and after 40 years of age [1, 2].

Genetics

The inheritance of psoriasis is quite complex, and does not fit into a simple recessive or dominant Mendelian inheritance pattern. Other factors, including environmental ones, may be involved. It is known that having a first-degree relative with psoriasis confers an increased risk of disease [3]. Psoriasis is a complex genetic disease, accounting for the difficulty in identifying susceptibility genes. What is known is that there are multiple susceptibility regions that have been identified, which contain genetic polymorphisms that confer an increased risk of developing psoriasis. The best characterized is PSORS1, in which HLA-Cw6 was recently identified as the definitive allele which confers the elevated risk [4, 5].

Pathogenesis

Psoriasis involves a complex interplay between various cells of the immune system and skin, including dermal dendritic cells, T cells, neutrophils, and keratinocytes. CD8+ T cells populate the epidermis, while macrophages, CD4+ T cells, and dermal dendritic cells reside in the superficial dermis. A multitude of cytokines, chemokines, and cell surface receptors are involved in a web of molecular pathways leading to clinical disease. Psoriasis is considered to be an immune-mediated disease characterized by a predominantly Th1-type cytokine profile in lesional skin with elevated levels of interferon-γ, TNF-α, IL-12, and IL-18, among others. More recently, the Th17 pathway has proven to be critical for maintenance of the chronic inflammatory process. At the center of this pathway is the CD4+ T cell, whose maintenance is supported by IL-23 secreted by antigen-presenting cells (dermal dendritic cells). These Th17 CD4+ T cells secrete IL-17 and IL-22, contributing to the enhancement and maintenance of inflammation and epidermal proliferation [6, 7].

Morphologic Subtypes

In its most classic morphologic presentation, psoriasis is characterized by red scaling elevated plaques. These correlate to the inflammation, vascular dilatation, and altered epidermal proliferation and differentiation (regular hyperplasia and hyperparakeratosis) seen histologically. Variations of this plaque morphology include red scaling patches (more often seen in the scalp, inverse, and erythrodermic forms of psoriasis) and the red scaling papules seen in early or flaring, guttate, or follicular psoriasis.

The second morphologic presentation is one of superficial pustules, characterized by intra-epidermal neutrophil accumulation with only mild epidermal hyperplasia on histology. Variations of this morphology include discrete and/or confluent superficial yellow-white pustules, either on a smooth erythematous edematous base or overlying normal-appearing skin (as seen in pustular psoriasis of von Zumbusch) or superficial discrete dirty yellow-brown pustules often found on the hands or feet (as seen in palmoplantar pustulosis).

Although there are 2 main morphologies, there are multiple subtypes of psoriasis that have been described based upon a combination of morphology, distribution, and pattern. These subtypes often occur alone. However, there may be an overlap or transition from one subtype to another due to various triggers or evolution of the disease. The subtypes are described in the following sections.

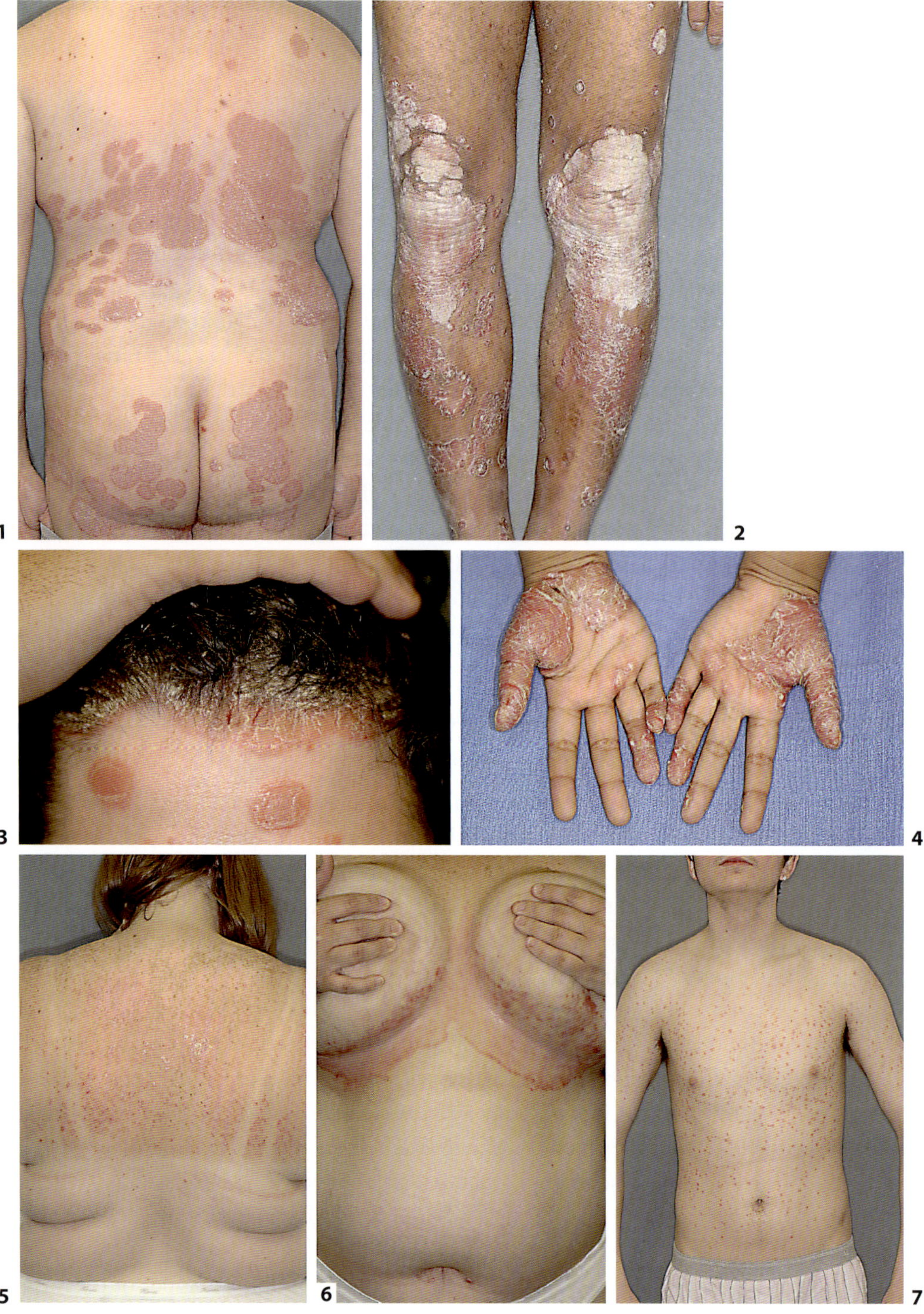

Fig. 1,2. Plaque psoriasis. Back and buttocks (**1**) and lower extremities (**2**) of two patients with plaque psoriasis, showing the variations in erythema, scale, and symmetry in this type of psoriasis.
Fig. 3. Scalp psoriasis. Extension of plaques onto the forehead in a patient with diffuse involvement of the scalp associated with focal hair thinning.

Plaque Psoriasis

This is the most common and well-recognized form of psoriasis. It is characterized by well-defined raised erythematous papules and plaques with silvery coarse scale. There can be great variation in the intensity of erythema (ranging from light pink to bright red to deep purplish red), elevation of the lesion (flat to very thick and elevated), and amount of scale (scattered light diffuse white scale overlying the lesion to thick micaceous hyperkeratotic scale in which the color and thickness of the lesion are not easily discernable; fig. 1, 2). The distribution is typically symmetric, and sites of predilection include the extensor surfaces of the extremities, particularly the elbows and knees, sacrum, scalp, nape of the neck, and to a lesser extent the remainder of the trunk, genitalia, face, and ears [8] (fig. 3). Individuals may present with hyperkeratotic scaling disease localized to the scalp only, making it difficult to discriminate from severe seborrheic dermatitis or tinea capitis. This presentation has been called tinea amiantacea, and requires evaluation to distinguish between these 3 entities. Plaque psoriasis localized to the palms and soles can have a significant impact on the patient's quality of life and function (fig. 4). At times, ill-defined or partially treated plaques localized only to the palms and soles can be difficult to distinguish from chronic hand dermatitis as both conditions can have erythema, scaling, fissuring, pain, itching, and nail changes. Biopsies are often equivocal and may suggest a psoriasiform dermatitis.

Additional features of psoriatic plaques include the Auspitz sign and Woronoff's ring. Auspitz sign is the presence of pinpoint bleeding at the base of a plaque after scale is forcibly removed. Its presence can sometimes be helpful, but it is not present in all cases and can also be seen in other disorders [9]. Woronoff's ring refers to the presence of a white ring around erythematous plaques undergoing topical treatment or phototherapy [10]. Interestingly, some patients develop lesions at sites of trauma, including those from sunburn. This phenomenon is known as the isomorphic or Köbner phenomenon (fig. 5).

Fig. 4. Palmar plaque psoriasis and psoriatic arthritis. This 10-year-old female has restricted use of her hands due to tightness, fissuring, itching, and pain. Note the flexion contracture of the 5th digit from psoriatic arthritis.

Fig. 5. Köbner phenomenon. A patient with a history of scalp psoriasis who developed lesions on the upper back 3 weeks following a sunburn to the area.

Fig. 6. Inverse psoriasis. Thin plaques localized to inframammary regions in a patient with psoriasis that also involved the axillary, inguinal, abdominal, and gluteal folds.

Fig. 7. Guttate psoriasis. Acute generalized scaly papules in a patient with asymptomatic streptococcus colonization of the pharynx.

Inverse Psoriasis

Inverse psoriasis is characterized mainly by its distribution: it is localized predominantly to intertriginous regions including the axillae, inframammary regions, gluteal cleft, genitals, abdominal folds and inguinal folds. These lesions also differ in morphology from that of typical plaque psoriasis lesions in that they are well-defined shiny erythematous patches or thin plaques without significant scale [6, 11] (fig. 6). The presentation may initially be confused for bacterial (often accentuated in the crease), candidal (appearance of superficial pustules and 1- to 2-mm superficial round erosions often helpful for diagnosis), or fungal intertrigo (less involvement of the crease, peripheral desquamative-type scale and possible fungal involvement elsewhere, such as the feet, gluteal cheeks, or toenails). Scrapings or cultures are sometimes needed to discriminate between these entities.

Guttate Psoriasis

This form of psoriasis is characterized by an acute generalized eruption of smaller round to oval-shaped well-defined erythematous scaly papules and plaques up to 1 cm in size [12] (fig. 7). This is considered to be more of an eruptive form of psoriasis and is often associated with infection, especially streptococcal pharyngitis [13]. More common in children and young adults, guttate psoriasis may initially respond well to antibiotics, heliotherapy, or phototherapy and go into remission, only to recur with reinfection.

Patients with guttate psoriasis may have a higher risk of developing plaque psoriasis later in life. On the other hand, for some patients, guttate psoriasis may be the initial manifestation of chronic psoriasis, triggered by infection or stress, only to evolve into the plaque-type over time. Guttate psoriasis can also be easily confused with the papular type of acutely flaring plaque psoriasis. The nature of the prior course, triggering factors, and intensity of erythema and scale (less in guttate) may help in differentiating these. Guttate psoriasis may also be confused with pityriasis rosea (PR), but differs in the nature of the scale (psoriatic scale involves the entire lesion and is more coarse, rather than the finer localized trailing ring pattern of the scale in PR), pattern (psoriasis does not present in a Christmas tree pattern and is less likely to appear in linear arrangements in the axilla and neck), and course (guttate psoriasis often lasts longer than 8 weeks unless appropriately treated, while PR often resolves within 6–8 weeks without treatment).

Although guttate psoriasis is highly associated with streptococcal infections, there is little evidence-based data, as documented in a Cochrane library review, to support treatment of these patients with antibiotics [14]. In the authors' experience, patients with an acute papular psoriatic eruption with a throat culture positive for streptococcus or markedly elevated antistreptolysin titers have a moderate chance of improving and sometimes clearing their psoriasis with oral antibiotics.

Erythrodermic Psoriasis

When involvement of psoriasis becomes so diffuse that it involves more than 90% of the total body surface area, a patient is considered to be erythrodermic. With confluence of the lesions and diffuse involvement, the lesions may be thinner or truly flat, and it may be difficult to identify lesions of classic plaque psoriasis. The skin may be warm to the touch due to increased perfusion, and the nature of erythema may vary depending on the patient's skin color and acuity of disease (brighter red with acuity or flaring). The scaling is also of a different quality; it is more fine, flaky, and desquamative rather than the typical silvery coarse thick scale of plaque psoriasis (fig. 8, 9). Of note, facial involvement may lead to ectropion.

Although not specific to erythrodermic psoriasis, as it can be seen in patients with erythroderma of any cause, associated clinical findings may include lymphadenopathy, fever or hypothermia, tachycardia, and peripheral edema. Associated laboratory findings can include an elevated erythrocyte sedimentation rate, hypoalbuminemia, leukocytosis or leukopenia, anemia, and elevations of lactate dehydrogenase, liver transaminases, uric acid, and calcium [15]. Precipitants for erythrodermic psoriasis include the tapering or discontinuation of systemic medications (such as corticosteroids, cyclosporine, or methotrexate), phototherapy-related toxicity, irritants (such as tar), and systemic illness or infection. Significant morbidity may occur due to dehydration from extensive fluid and electrolyte disturbances, protein losses, high-output cardiac failure, and infection.

Psoriasis is only one of many causes of erythroderma. Cutaneous T cell lymphoma – typically in the setting of Sezary syndrome, atopic dermatitis, drug reactions, other papulosquamous skin diseases (such as pityriasis rubra pilaris), as well as connective tissue diseases such as lupus or dermatomyositis among others – can also present as exfoliative erythroderma. Presence of classic cutaneous, scalp, or inverse lesions, nail findings, or personal or family history of psoriasis may provide clues to the etiology of erythroderma [16]. Skin biopsies are often unhelpful in confirming erythroderma secondary to psoriasis, but may be helpful in ruling out cutaneous T cell lymphoma or connective tissue disease.

Small Plaque Psoriasis

This form of psoriasis is similar in morphology to guttate psoriasis with discrete papules and plaques, with lesions as large as 3 cm in size. However, small plaque psoriasis represents a chronic form of psoriasis rather than an acute eruptive process [12]. This variant may not have the pattern of accentuation on the extensor extremities, scalp, elbows, and knees as in classic psoriasis, and may have a more randomly distributed, scattered, and diffuse pattern.

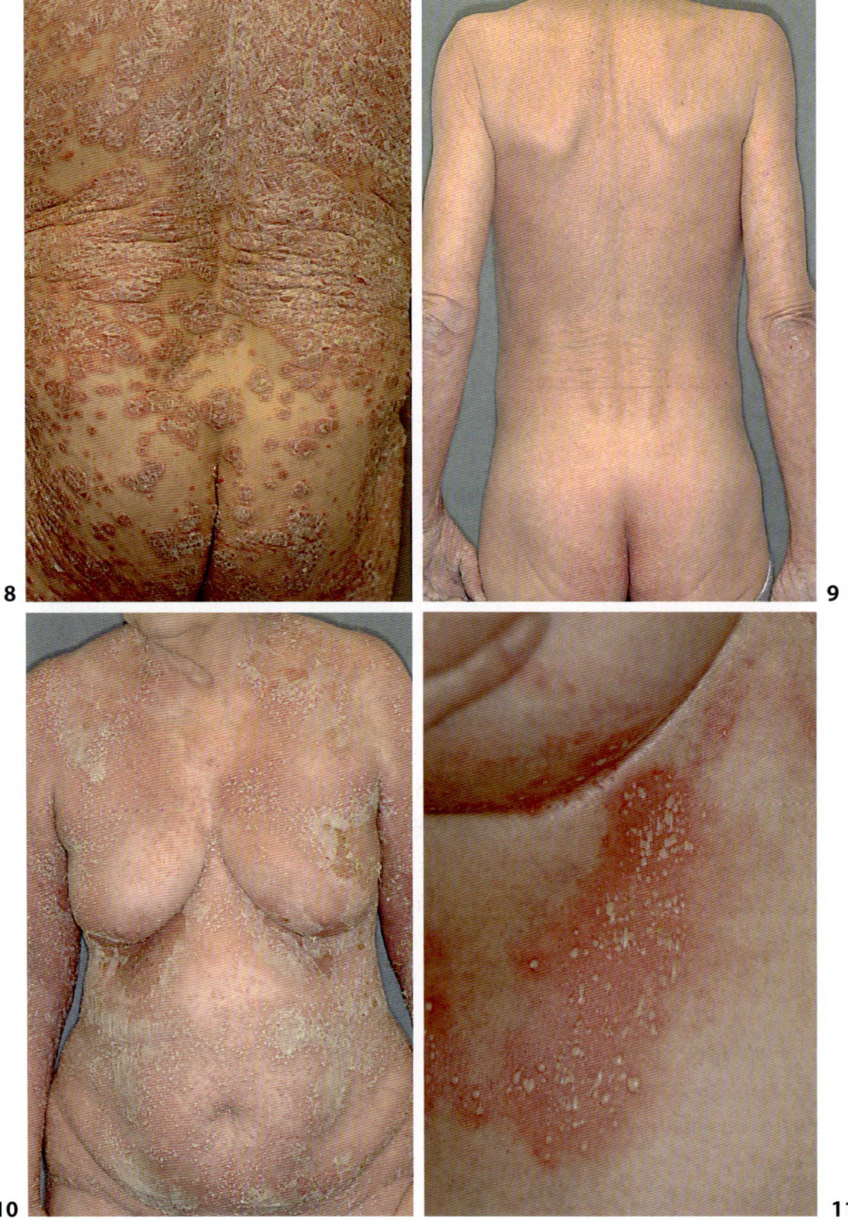

Fig. 8, 9. 8 Extensive or generalized plaque psoriasis. **9** Erythrodermic psoriasis. Generalized erythema and fine scaling characteristic of erythroderma. The classic plaque psoriasis lesions on the elbows (pictured), as well as classic scalp and nail involvement helped differentiate this erythrodermic patient from other causes of erythroderma.

Fig. 10, 11. Pustular psoriasis of von Zumbusch. Recurrent generalized erythematous edematous patches studded with discrete and confluent pustules requiring multiple hospitalizations, at normal (**10**) and higher magnifications (**11**). Evaluation for immunobullous disorders and medication-induced acute generalized exanthematic pustulosis was unremarkable. The patient required combination acitretin, methotrexate, and infliximab for adequate control.

Pustular Psoriasis

Generalized Psoriasis

Also known as von Zumbusch psoriasis, this rare form of psoriasis is characterized by the rapid development of widespread tender erythema followed by an eruption of 1- to 2-mm pustules (fig. 10, 11). The skin eruption is generally preceded or accompanied by fever and malaise. Leukocytosis and elevated ESR are commonly encountered. This severe form of psoriasis carries an increased morbidity and mortality (stemming from risk of secondary bacterial and fungal superinfections) and, rarely, acute respiratory distress syndrome. Precipitants have included infections, medications, decreased dose of systemic steroids, and UV exposure, among others [17–19]. Urgent treatment with systemic medications is required and hospitalization should be strongly considered if the condition is rapidly evolving.

Localized Forms

This form describes the development of pustules locally, within established plaques of psoriasis (indicating unstable disease) or pustules alone, either discretely or in confluence. The pustular form of psoriasis may occur anywhere preexisting or new plaques are developing. A second variant includes pustular psoriasis of the hands and feet, and includes 2 subtypes: acrodermatitis continua of Hallopeau and pustulosis palmaris et plantaris (palmar/plantar pustulosis). The latter 2 subtypes are similar in that they are generally chronic, resistant to therapy, and present a challenge to the treating physician. In the palmoplantar variant, pruritic or burning erythematous patches are distributed on the palms and soles, within which develop multiple 2- to 5-mm pustules, the early ones of which are yellow and the older ones are brown (fig. 12). In acrodermatitis, erythema, scaling, and pustules develop at the tips of the fingers or toes (usually a single digit) and progress proximally to involve and ultimately destroy the nail bed and matrix [20] (fig. 13, 14).

Annular Psoriasis

Annular pustular psoriasis is a distinct variant that is characterized by a subacute onset of hyperpigmented to erythematous plaques with peripheral pustules. It can, however, also present within the context of generalized pustular psoriasis. Interestingly, a greater proportion of cases of pustular psoriasis in children are of this subtype compared to adults. The course may be characterized by recurrences, and the severity is generally less intense than that of generalized pustular psoriasis (von Zumbusch) [21, 22].

Pustular Psoriasis of Pregnancy

This rare form of pustular psoriasis is also known as impetigo herpetiformis. Characteristic to this form of psoriasis is its association with pregnancy and its resolution with delivery. Morphologically, the lesions are erythematous patches or plaques

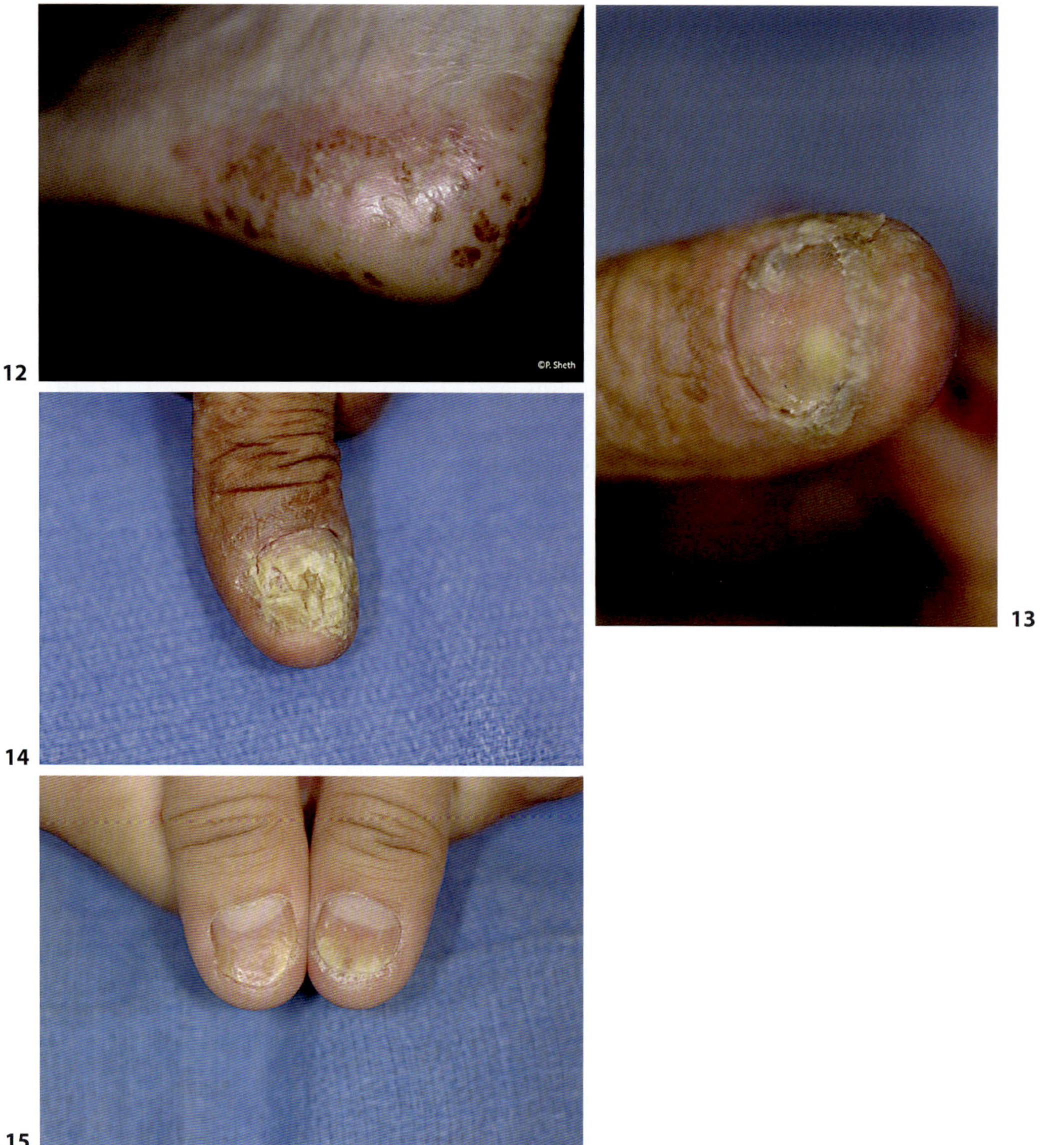

Fig. 12. Palmoplantar pustular psoriasis. Circumscribed erythema of the heel within which are multiple yellow pustules and older brown papules characteristic of this form of psoriasis.

Fig. 13, 14. Acrodermatitis continua of Hallopeau. **13** Early-stage pustular psoriasis localized to the distal thumb. **14** Erythema, crusting, and subungual pustules resulted in complete dystrophy of the nail within 3 months.

Fig. 15. Nail psoriasis. Distal onycholysis, pitting, and oil drop sign in a patient with plaque psoriasis and psoriatic arthritis.

with peripheral pustules that initially begin in flexural areas and ultimately generalize. Patients are often affected earlier in their course of pregnancy and more severely with subsequent pregnancies. Increased fetal mortality is an important complication. There have also been reports of recurrences following pregnancy but associated with monthly menses and oral contraceptives [23–26].

Nail Psoriasis

A multitude of nail findings can present with psoriasis. Individually, these findings or signs may not be specific to psoriasis; however, the more of these findings found in the nail, the more specific it is for psoriasis. Nail pitting is a relatively common finding, but can be found with other diseases such as eczema, alopecia areata, and lichen planus. It is characterized by small round depressions within the surface of the nail plate and represents involvement of the nail matrix. Other signs of nail psoriasis include the salmon patch or oil drop sign indicating nail bed involvement, onycholysis representing distal separation of the nail plate from the nail bed, white silvery subungual hyperkeratosis, red spots in the lunula representing dilated tortuous vessels associated with psoriasis, leukonychia, vertical or transverse ridging, and, finally, nail bed hemorrhages (fig. 15). With severe involvement the nail may diffusely crumble and ultimately detach [27]. Nail psoriasis may have a notable impact on quality of life of some individuals, as it can impact the functionality of the hands for hobbies, work, and everyday living. In addition, it important to screen patients for nail psoriasis as it has been shown that psoriatic nail disease (along with scalp psoriasis and intergluteal psoriasis) is associated with a higher likelihood of psoriatic arthritis [28].

Oral Manifestations

Patients with psoriasis may also present with oral findings. Geographic tongue (benign migratory glossitis), characterized by geographic patterns of erythematous patches surrounded by a white line and loss of filiform papillae on the dorsum of the tongue (fig. 16), and fissured tongue, characterized by deep longitudinal fissures, are the forms most commonly encountered. However, it is important to note that individuals without psoriasis can also display these findings, but it is thought to be at a lower rate than individuals with psoriasis [29]. Some studies have found no correlation between this condition, and others report a high occurrence [30, 31]. In the authors' experience in the psoriasis clinic in Cincinnati (Ohio, USA), the prevalence of geographic tongue in patients with plaque psoriasis is uncommon (less than 5%).

Special Population: Children

Affected children can present with morphologies similar to those found in adults [for detailed information on psoriasis in children, see 'Therapy of childhood psoriasis' by Trüeb, R.M.]. Plaque psoriasis, plaque psoriasis isolated to the scalp, guttate psoriasis, and inverse psoriasis are commonly encountered. Palmoplantar, pustular, and nail forms are less commonly encountered. Psoriasiform diaper dermatitis with disseminated lesions on the trunk represents a common form of presentation, particularly in children under the age of 2 years [32, 33]. It is not uncommon to see children diagnosed with 'chronic eczema' of the scalp, ears, fingers, or other areas, only later in childhood or adolescence to have the condition evolve into plaque psoriasis of more typical appearance. One of the clues to the diagnosis of psoriasis early in childhood is the distribution (scalp, medial upper eyelids, perinasal, ears, intertriginous, genitalia, nails being more common) and the relative lack of pruritus of these more eczematous-appearing patches.

Course

The course of the disease, particularly plaque psoriasis, is chronic with periodic remissions of variable duration occasionally lasting years (without therapy). [8] In the authors' experience, guttate psoriasis can become chronic and take on the features of chronic plaque psoriasis or in some cases resolve with treatment of the inciting infection, only to recur again in the future with precipitating events. The primary form of generalized and localized pustular psoriasis is also chronic, with periodic remissions. Secondary forms of pustular psoriasis, in the setting of plaque psoriasis, may be transient or become the new morphology after conversion. This may be seen as well in erythrodermic psoriasis (differentiated from generalized plaque psoriasis); it may be transient (weeks, months, or a few years) in duration or chronic (less often).

Triggering Factors

Initiation or exacerbation of psoriasis has been ascribed to multiple triggers. Environment, such as a change in climate with lower temperatures, humidity, and sunlight may play a role in the winter flares of patients from colder climates. Physical and psychological stress may be key exacerbating factors for psoriasis [34].

Other trigger factors include infection (strep, HIV), traumatic injury to the skin, surgery involving the skin, drugs such as lithium and β-blockers, smoking, and excessive alcohol intake [35].

Laboratory Findings

A variety of laboratory abnormalities can be encountered with psoriasis, particularly with erythroderma (as discussed in 'Erythrodermic psoriasis'). In addition, with the increasing association of obesity and other comorbidities with psoriasis, abnormalities in liver enzymes, lipid profile, and glucose tolerance may be increased in some psoriatic patients. There are multiple ongoing long-term pharmaceutical registry studies evaluating some of these issues. Awaiting conclusive data, the authors currently obtain baseline liver function studies, fasting lipid profile, metabolic profile, C-reactive protein measurements, tuberculosis screening (purified protein derivative test and/or chest X-ray, as indicated), hepatitis B and C virus screening, and complete blood count in patients with moderate to severe psoriasis who are candidates for systemic therapy. This is helpful in screening for some of the comorbidities associated with psoriasis, as well as for assessing the appropriateness of various systemic therapies.

Comorbidities

The effects of psoriasis extend beyond cutaneous involvement, and are associated with other organ systems as well [for detailed information on comorbidities, see 'Impact of comorbidities on the management of psoriasis' by Gerdes, S. and Mrowietz, U.].

Psoriatic arthritis affects a significant proportion of patients with psoriasis, although its true incidence is unclear with reports ranging from 6 to 42% [36]. Its incidence varies depending on the population being studied or surveyed, but likely averages around 15–20% of the psoriatic population. Psoriatic arthritis is included among the inflammatory arthropathies with potential for severe joint destruction without proper management. Its presence has implications for medical management, and deserves appropriate radiological studies and evaluation if suspected.

Recently, it has been shown that patients with psoriasis are more likely to have traditional cardiovascular risk factors, such as hyperlipidemia, hypertension, diabetes, obesity, tobacco use, and a history of previous myocardial infarction. In addition, evidence has suggested that psoriasis is an independent risk factor for myocardial infarction when controlling for the aforementioned risk factors. Interestingly, the risk remained elevated despite excluding patients treated with medications that elevate lipids and blood pressure, specifically retinoids and cyclosporine [37–39].

Patients with psoriasis have also been shown to have a slightly increased likelihood of having lymphoma compared to individuals without psoriasis. The association has been reported to be greater with cutaneous T cell lymphomas and Hodgkin lymphoma, and inconsistent with non-Hodgkin lymphoma [40–42].

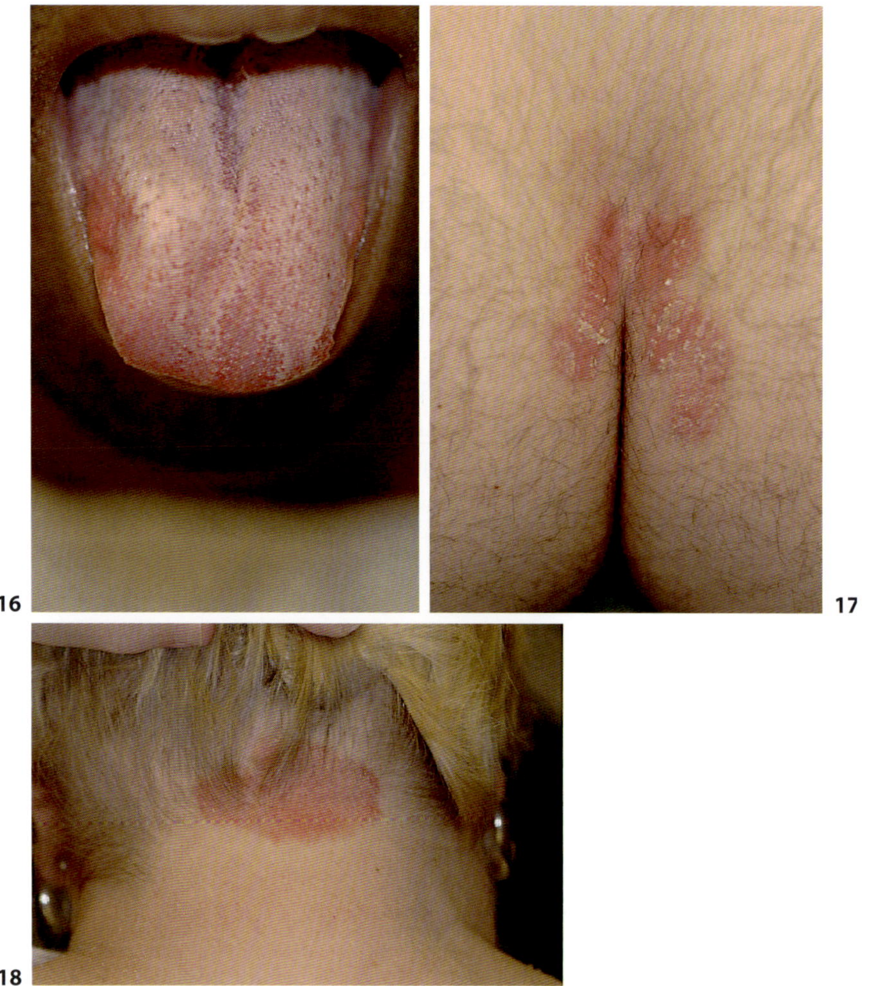

Fig. 16. Geographic and fissured tongue. Mild annular and arciform changes of the tongue and a mid-dorsal tongue fissure.
Fig. 17, 18. Skin clues to psoriatic arthritis. Asymptomatic solitary plaque of the superior gluteal cleft (**17**) and the posterior scalp (**18**) as the only manifestation of psoriasis in 2 patients with psoriatic arthritis. A full skin, nail, and scalp examination is recommended in patients with inflammatory arthritis or spondyloarthropathy.

Finally, psoriasis can have a dramatic impact on social, professional, and personal relationships. Its presence may lead to problems with anxiety and depression, often leading to a negative impact on treatment due to mistrust, apathy or non-compliance. These issues necessitate a high index of suspicion by the treating physician so that appropriate treatment or referral may ensue.

Table 1. Differential diagnosis of psoriasis

Chronic dermatitis
Seborrheic dermatitis
Pityriasis rosea
Other papulosquamous disorders (including pityriasis rubra pilaris, pityriasis lichenoides chronica, and lichen planus)
Mycosis fungoides
Syphilis
Cutaneous lupus
Intertrigo (candidal, fungal, bacterial)
Other pustular eruptions (acute generalized exanthematous pustulosis, varicella, disseminated herpes simplex or zoster, extensive bacterial folliculitis)
Localized pustular eruptions (herpetic whitlow, folliculitis, scabies)

Differential Diagnosis

Classic presentations of psoriasis are infrequently confused with other conditions (table 1). However, atypical presentations or lesions other than the classic plaque form of psoriasis can present a diagnostic challenge. Clues to final clinical diagnosis often hinge on a complete skin examination (searching the distribution to rule out involvement of the superior gluteal cleft, posterior scalp, umbilicus, elbows, knees, or inverse areas for involvement), 1 or more skin biopsies if necessary, other symptoms (if psoriasis is asymptomatic) and evolution (fig. 17, 18).

The presence of psoriasis with sole scalp involvement may be difficult to discern from severe seborrheic dermatitis, even for the expert. In the authors' experience, patients with dry white adherent scale of the scalp, even when suggestive of seborrheic dermatitis on distribution, often develop scalp psoriasis over time. Chronic lichenified eczematous lesions on the extremities may also appear morphologically similar to lesions of chronic plaque psoriasis. Looking for other clues, as previously mentioned, as well as symmetry, nail pitting, or geographic tongue in addition to a family history of psoriasis may help in establishing an accurate diagnosis. When considering a diagnosis of guttate psoriasis, one must also consider pityriasis rosea (arranged in the lines of cleavage) and syphilis (generally has involvement of the palms and soles and a history of previous painless oral or genital chancre). Predominant involvement of flexural areas may lead some practitioners to suspect candidal, bacterial, or fungal intertrigo. The presence of brightly erythematous papules, pustules and satellite lesions at the periphery should provide clues for a candidal etiology. Central clearing and peripheral scaling should prompt a potassium hydroxide examination of scale for dermatophyte forms. Pustular variants of psoriasis may be readily diagnosed in an individual with either current or previous classic lesions of psoriasis. However, if the clinical situation is uncertain, performing bacterial or viral cultures in addition to biopsy may be indicated to rule out infectious diseases.

Severity of Psoriasis

It has been anecdotally reported that approximately 75–83% of patients with psoriasis have mild involvement, and that 17–25% have moderate or severe involvement [43]. However, there is no uniformly accepted definition or guidelines for the severity of psoriasis. In addition, the severity of psoriasis varies over the time course of the disease and an individual may have 'severe disease' at one time in his or her life and 'mild' disease at another time. The determination of severity is important in classifying patients for study purposes, for society to measure the economic impact of psoriasis, and for helping direct guidelines and decision-making in determining the course of therapy.

The severity of psoriasis in the clinical setting has been measured using various tools over the years. Of these, the 2 most common measurements in practice are the percentage of body surface area (BSA) involved, either measured by the full hand print (in which the palm and digits equal approximately 1% BSA) or the 'rule of 9's' (in which different regions of the body are equal to 9% or a multiple of 9% of the BSA), and the global severity of the skin lesions or global disease (which takes into account the depth of erythema, magnitude of plaque elevation, and amount of scale).

For research purposes, multiple scales have been developed to incorporate the measurement of these variables into objective, reliable, and reproducible scores [44]. Measurements such as the Psoriasis Area and Severity Index (PASI) and Physician's Global Assessment (PGA) represent the most common ones used in the current clinical research studies for moderate to severe psoriasis [for more detailed information, see 'Topical treatment of psoriasis' by Kamili Q.u.A. and Menter A.].

The appreciation and importance of how psoriasis impacts the quality of life of the individual, and therefore its impact on the overall severity of the disease, has led to the use of multiple questionnaire-based measures [SKINDEX, Dermatology Life Quality Index (DQLI), Psoriasis Disability Index, Psoriasis Life Stress Inventory, Psoriasis Quality of Life Questionnaire, and Psoriasis Quality of Life 12-Item Questionnaire) to help better define psoriasis severity [45, 46]. Of these, the most common quality of life measure used in clinical trials is the DLQI [47].

A combination of these measures has been used to identify patients with moderate to severe psoriasis for inclusion into studies of biologic agents. The criteria of BSA greater than or equal to 10% and/or a PASI of greater than or equal to 10 or 12 have been minimum criteria for inclusion into these. This does not however suggest that a BSA of 10% is accepted as moderate, as previously defined by the US FDA in which 10% BSA was moderate and 20% was severe. It has been suggested that the rule of '10's' be considered in guiding the use of biologic therapies (in some countries

Table 2. National Psoriasis Foundation's recommendations for localized vs. systemic or photo(chemo) therapy

Candidates for localized therapies	Candidates for systemic or photo(chemo)therapy
Less than 5% BSA	Greater than 5% BSA, or less than 5% BSA with involvement of scalp, face, genitals, nails, palms/soles Erythrodermic psoriasis Pustular psoriasis Guttate psoriasis Resistance to localized therapy Significant physical or mental disability

reserved for 'severe psoriasis'). In this rule, the score of 10 or more for either the PASI, the BSA, or the DLQI would indicate severe disease, and therefore, along with other criteria, justify the use of the biologic therapy.

The National Psoriasis Foundation's Clinical Consensus on Disease Severity [48], in developing recommendations on selecting treatment for plaque psoriasis, suggested a change in the traditional paradigm of labeling patients as mild, moderate, or severe. Instead, the consensus statement proposed a 2-tiered system for plaque psoriasis that reflected how patients in the US were being treated in clinical practice. Although aligned with the model of determining if a patient is mild or moderate-severe, the recommendation was to determine if the patient is a candidate for localized treatment vs. phototherapy/systemic treatment based on a combination of criteria (table 2). These criteria are more easily applied in the clinical practice setting, and do not require the use of more time-intensive tools.

In the authors' practice, a decision for the use of localized therapies, such as topical agents, excimer laser, or intralesional steroids vs. systemic (traditional or biologic) therapy or photo(chemo)therapy, is based on a variety of factors. The type of psoriasis (guttate, pustular, plaque, palmar/plantar, etc.), the presence of psoriatic arthritis, a BSA of greater than 5%, and a global disease severity of moderate redness, thickness, and scaling (if plaque type) would be part of the initial criteria for consideration of systemic therapy or phototherapy.

However, just as important would be the patient's own assessment of his or her disease severity, the type and location of psoriasis, the impact on the patient's quality of life (either upon direct discussion of its impact or through a validated tool such as the DLQI), history of failed prior therapies, history of severe or unstable disease, course of disease (slowly or rapidly progressing, presence of triggers), life situation (family planning, type of work, access and affordability of care, etc.), and the presence or increased risk of comorbidities. In addition, if topical or localized therapies, when used appropriately, have not been effective in improving the psoriasis or the quality of life of the individual, systemic or photo(chemo)therapy should be considered.

Indications for Referral

Referral to a dermatologist should be considered when a diagnosis is suspected but not certain. Skin biopsy and interpretation by a dermatopathologist can greatly aid in confirming the diagnosis. Any patient with psoriasis that has a moderate to severe impact on their quality of life (physical, work, emotional, social, marital, etc), pediatric patients with moderate to severe psoriasis, patients with moderate to severe psoriasis requiring phototherapy or systemic therapy, psoriasis that involves sensitive areas (inverse, face and scalp, palms and soles), and psoriasis that is unresponsive to first-line therapies (topical steroids, tars, vitamin D or A analogues, sunlight therapy) should be considered for referral to a specialist familiar with systemic medications and phototherapy. In addition, patients with comorbidities, including psoriatic arthritis, that affect treatment considerations should be considered for referral.

In the same fashion, patients with moderate to severe psoriasis, due to the possible higher risk of cardiovascular disease, obesity and metabolic syndrome, depression, psoriatic arthritis, and other associated comorbidities, should be considered for referral by the dermatologist to the internist/general practitioner to evaluate and manage these comorbidities. As we learn more about psoriasis as being more than a disease affecting just the skin, partnership of the different disciplines of medicine will afford the best care for the patient with psoriatic disease.

References

1 Gudjonsson JE, Elder JT: Psoriasis: epidemiology. Clin Dermatol 2007;25:535–546.
2 Gelfand JM, Stern RS, Nijsten T, Feldman SR, Thoma J, Kist J, Rolstad T, Margolis DJ: The prevalence of psoriasis in African Americans: results from a population-based study. J Am Acad Dermatol 2005;52:23–26.
3 Swanbeck G, Inerot A, Martinsson T, Wahlstrom J: A population genetic study of psoriasis. Acta Derm Venereol Suppl (Stockh) 1994;186:7–8.
4 Elder JT: PSORS1: linking genetics and immunology. J Invest Dermatol 2006;126:1205–1206.
5 Nair RP, Stuart PE, Nistor I, Hiremagalore R, Chia NVC, Jenisch S, Weichenthal M, Abecasis GR, Lim HW, Christophers E, Voorhees JJ, Elder JT: Sequence and haplotype analysis supports *HLA-C* as the psoriasis susceptibility 1 gene. Am J Hum Genetics 2006;78:827–851.
6 Wolff K, Goldsmith LA, Katz SI, Gilchrest BA, Paller AS, Leffell DJ: Fitzpatrick's Dermatology in General Medicine, ed 7. New York, McGraw Hill, 2008, vol 1, pp 170–179.
7 Lowes MA, Bowcock AM, Krueger JG: Pathogenesis and therapy of psoriasis. Nature 2007;445:866–873.
8 Farber EM, Nall ML: The natural history of psoriasis in 5,600 patients. Dermatologica 1974;148:1–18.
9 Bernhard JD: Auspitz sign is not sensitive or specific for psoriasis. J Am Acad Dermatol 1990;22(part 1):1079–1081.
10 Penneys NS, Ziboh V, Simon P: Pathogenesis of Woronoff ring in psoriasis. Arch Dermatol 1976; 112:955–957.
11 Wang G, Li C, Gao T, Liu Y: Clinical analysis of 48 cases of inverse psoriasis: a hospital-based study. Eur J Dermatol 2005;15:176–178.

12 Griffiths CEM, Christophers E, Barker JNWN, Chalmers RJG, Chimenti S, Krueger GG, Leonardi C, Menter A, Ortonne JP, Fry L: A classification of psoriasis vulgaris according to phenotype. Br J Dermatol 2007;156:258–262.

13 Telfer NR, Chalmers RJG, Whale K, Colman G: The role of streptococcal infection in the initiation of guttate psoriasis. Arch Dermatol 1992;128:39–42.

14 Owen CM, Chalmers R, O'Sullivan T, Griffiths CEM: Antistreptococcal interventions for guttate and chronic plaque psoriasis. Cochrane Database Syst Rev 2000;2:CD001976. DOI: 10.1002/14651858.CD001976.

15 Boyd AS, Menter A: Erythrodermic psoriasis: precipitating factors, course, and prognosis in 50 patients. J Am Acad Dermatol 1989;21(part 1):985–991.

16 Rothe MJ, Bialy TL, Grant-Kels JM: Erythroderma. Dermatol Clin 2000;18:405–415.

17 Zelickson BD, Muller SA: Generalized pustular psoriasis. Arch Dermatol 1991;127:1339–1345.

18 Abou-Samra T, Constantin JM, Amarger S, Mansard S, Souteyrand P, Bazin JE, D'Incan M: Generalized pustular psoriasis complicated by acute respiratory distress syndrome. Br J Dermatol 2004;150:353–356.

19 Baker H, Ryan TJ: Generalized pustular psoriasis: a clinical and epidemiological study of 104 cases. Br J Dermatol 1968;80:771–793.

20 Rook A, Champion JL, Burton JL, Wilkinson DS, Burns DA, Ebling FJG, Breathnach SM: Rook/Wilkinson/Ebling Textbook of Dermatology, ed 6. London, Blackwell Science, 1998, vol 2, pp 1633–1636.

21 Liao PB, Rubinson R, Howard R, Sanchez G, Frieden IJ: Annular pustular psoriasis – most common form of pustular psoriasis in children: report of 3 cases and review of the literature. Pediatr Dermatol 2002; 19:19–25.

22 Rosen RM: Annular pustular psoriasis induced by UV radiation from tanning salon use. J Am Acad Dermatol 1991;25(part 1):336–337.

23 Chaidemenos G, Lefaki I, Tsakiri A, Mourellou O: Impetigo herpetiformis: menstrual exacerbations for 7 years postpartum. Eur Acad Dermatol Venereol 2005;19:466–469.

24 Breier-Maly J, Ortel B, Breier F, Schmidt JB, Honigsmann H: Generalized pustular psoriasis of pregnancy (impetigo herpetiformis). Dermatology 1999;198:61–64.

25 Oumeish OY, Farraj SE, Bataineh AS: Some aspects of impetigo herpetiformis. 1982;118:103–105.

26 Lotem ML, Katzenelson V, Rotem A, Hod M, Sandbank M: Impetigo herpetiformis: a variant of pustular psoriasis or a separate entity? J Am Acad Dermatol 1989;20(part 2):338–341.

27 Jiaravuthisan MM, Sasseville D, Vender RB, Murphy F, Muhn CY: Psoriasis of the nail: anatomy, pathology, clinical presentation, and a review of the literature on therapy. J Am Acad Dermatol 2007;57: 1–27.

28 Wilson FC, Icen M, Crowson CS, McEvoy MT, Gabriel SE, Kremers HM: Incidence and clinical predictors of psoriatic arthritis in patients with psoriasis: a population-based study. Arthritis Rheum 2009;61:233–239.

29 Zhu JF, Kaminski MJ, Pulitzer DR, Hu J, Thomas HF: Psoriasis: pathophysiology and oral manifestations. Oral Dis 1996;2:135–144.

30 Hernandez-Perez F, Jaimes-Aveldanez A, Urquizo-Ruvalcaba Mde L, Diaz-Barcelot M, Irigoyen-Camacho ME, Vega-Memije ME, Mosqueda-Taylor A: Prevalence of oral lesions in patients with psoriasis. Med Oral Patol Oral Cir Bucal 2008;13: E703–E708.

31 Miloglu O, Goregen M, Akgul HM, Acemoglu H: The prevalence and risk factors associated with benign migratory glossitis lesions in 7,619 Turkish dental outpatients. Oral Surg Oral Med Oral Pathol Oral Radiol Endod 2009;107:e29–e33.

32 Morris AM, Rogers M, Fischer G, Williams K: Childhood psoriasis: a clinical review of 1,262 cases. Pediatr Dermatol 2001;18:188–198.

33 Seyhan M, Coskun BK, Saglam H, Ozcan H, Karincaoglu Y: Psoriasis in childhood and adolescence: evaluation of demographic and clinical features. Pediatr Int 2006;48:525–530.

34 Malhotra SK, Mehta V: Role of stressful life events in induction or exacerbation of psoriasis and chronic urticaria. Indian J Dermatol Venereol Leprol 2008; 74:594–599.

35 Dika E, Bardazzi F, Balestri R, Maibach HI: Environmental factors and psoriasis. Curr Probl Dermatol 2007;35:118–135.

36 Gottlieb A, Korman NJ, Gordon KB, Feldman SR, Lebwohl M, Koo JY, Van Voorhees AS, Elmets CA, Leonardi CL, Beutner KR, Bhushan R, Menter A: Guidelines of care for the management of psoriasis and psoriatic arthritis. 2. Psoriatic arthritis: overview and guidelines of care for treatment with an emphasis on the biologics. J Am Acad Dermatol 2008;58: 851–864.

37 Gelfand JM, Neimann AL, Shin DB: Risk of myocardial infarction in patients with psoriasis. JAMA 2006;296:1735–1741.

38 Kaye JA, Li L, Jick SS: Incidence of risk factors for myocardial infarction and other vascular disease in patient with psoriasis. Br J Dermatol 2008;159:895–902.

39 Neimann AL, Shin DB, Wang X, Margolis DJ, Troxel AB, Gelfand JM: Prevalence of cardiovascular risk factors in patients with psoriasis. J Am Acad Dermatol 2006;55:829–835.
40 Gelfand JM, Shin DB, Neimann AL, Wang X, Margolis DJ, Troxel AB: The risk of lymphoma in patients with psoriasis. J Invest Dermatol 2006;126: 2194–2201.
41 Smedby KE, Vajdic CM, Falster M, et al: Autoimmune disorders and risk of non-Hodgkin lymphoma subtypes: a pooled analysis within the InterLymph Consortium. Blood 2008;111:4029–4038.
42 Mellemkjaer L, Pfeiffer RM, Engels EA, Gridley G, Wheeler W, Hemminki K, Olsen JH, Dreyer L, Linet MS, Goldin LR, Landgren O: Autoimmune disease in individuals and close family members and susceptibility to non-Hodgkin's lymphoma. Arthritis Rheum 2008;58:657–666.
43 Kurd SK, Gelfand JM: The prevalence of previously diagnosed and undiagnosed psoriasis in US adults: results from NHANES 2003–2004. J Am Acad Dermatol 2009;60:218–224.
44 Berth-Jones J, Grotzinger K, Rainville C, Pham B, Huang J, Daly S, Herdman M, Firth P, Hotchkiss K: A study examining inter- and intrarater reliability of three scales for measuring severity of psoriasis: Psoriasis Area and Severity Index, Physician's Global Assessment and Lattice System Physician's Global Assessment. Br J Dermatol 2006;155:707–713.
45 McKenna SP, Cook SA, Whalley D, Doward LC, Richards HL, Griffiths CEM, Assche ADV: Development of the PSORI, a psoriasis-specific measure of quality of life designed for use in clinical practice and trials. Br J Dermatol 2003;149:323–331.
46 Menter A, Gottlieb A, Feldman SR, Van Voorhees AS, Leonardi CL, Gordon KB, Lebwohl M, Koo JYM, Elmets CA, Korman NJ, Beutner KR, Bhushan R: Guidelines of care for the management of psoriasis and psoriatic arthritis. 1. Overview of psoriasis and guidelines of care for the treatment of psoriasis with biologics. J Am Acad Dermatol 2008;58:826–850.
47 Gardune J, Bhosle MJ, Balkrishnan R, Feldman SR: Measures used in specifying psoriasis lesion(s), global disease and quality of life: a systematic review. J Dermatol Treat 2007;18:223–242.
48 Pariser DM, Bagel J, Gelfand JM, Korman NJ, Ritchlin CT, Strober BE, Van Voorhees AS, Young M, Rittenberg S, Lebwohl MG, Horn EJ: National psoriasis foundation clinical consensus on disease severity. Arch Dermatol 2007;143:239–242.

Pranav B. Sheth, MD
Group Health Associates
Clifton, 2915 Clifton Avenue
Cincinnati, Ohio 45220 (USA)
Tel. +1 513 872 2063, Fax +1 513 872 2068, E-Mail pranav.sheth1@yahoo.com

Yawalkar N (ed): Management of Psoriasis.
Curr Probl Dermatol. Basel, Karger, 2009, vol 38, pp 21–36

Impact of Comorbidities on the Management of Psoriasis

S. Gerdes · U. Mrowietz

Psoriasis-Center at the Department of Dermatology, University Medical Center Schleswig-Holstein, Campus Kiel, Kiel, Germany

Abstract

Psoriasis is associated with numerous comorbidities that have a major impact on severely affected patients. Besides psoriatic arthritis, other diseases such as metabolic syndrome and cardiovascular diseases are becoming of major importance. In particular, patients with severe forms of psoriasis are at a higher risk of developing cardiovascular diseases and myocardial infarction. In a recent study, a reduction in life expectancy was shown for this subgroup of patients. An increased prevalence of concomitant diseases leads to an increased intake of concomitant medication; thus, it is easy for comorbidities and their treatments to interact with routinely used antipsoriatic therapies and complicate the management of severely affected patients. This patient subgroup has a strong need of sufficient treatment not only for their severe skin symptoms, but also for preventing the possible development of comorbidities and their long-term complications. As dermatologists are often one of the first and most often consulted health care specialists for patients with psoriasis, advanced knowledge of the comorbid state of these patients should influence clinical management and lead to new standards of care. This article will summarize the current knowledge on comorbidities in psoriasis and their impact on patient management.

Psoriasis belongs to the group of immune-mediated inflammatory disorders (IMIDs) together with rheumatoid arthritis and inflammatory bowl disease (Crohn's disease) among others. Besides the skin manifestations, numerous studies have proven that there is an association between psoriasis and other concomitant diseases, referred to in the following as comorbidities. The best-known comorbidity is psoriatic arthritis (PsA), but other diseases, particularly metabolic syndrome and cardiovascular diseases (CVD), are becoming more important. The presence of comorbidities may influence the treatment options for psoriasis, either by contraindications for antipsoriatic medications or by interaction of comedications with systemic antipsoriatic treatment. Thus, the increased knowledge of comorbidities in this patient group has led to changes in standards of care. In the following, comorbidities and their impact on the treatment and management of patients with psoriasis will be discussed.

What Do We Know about Comorbidities of Patients with Psoriasis?

Psoriatic Arthritis

An association of rheumatic diseases with psoriasis was first described in the 19th century. In 1973, the occurrence of joint disorders in psoriasis patients was classified as a specific entity with distinct patterns, including the absence of rheumatoid factor and the presence of clinical characteristics such as an equal distribution between males and females, an asymmetric involvement of small peripheral joints, dactylitis, arthritis mutilans and ankylosing spondylitis. Today, PsA is classified among the spondylarthropathies, a cluster of diseases that share common features, such as absence of rheumatoid factor, axial involvement and an association with HLA-B27. An association of HLA-B27 and PsA is present in about 40–50% of patients. As this genetic marker is present in about 8% of the healthy white population, of whom 90% will never develop any form of spondylarthropathy, routine testing for HLA-B27 might not be clinically helpful [1]. A clinical hallmark of PsA is the involvement of ligaments and tendons, known as enthesopathy or enthesitis. In the majority of cases, the onset of PsA follows skin manifestations – even so in some cases PsA may precede skin lesions, which can complicate the diagnosis. Psoriatic nail involvement is more common in patients with PsA than in patients without PsA. The clinical course of PsA is usually independent of the course of skin symptoms, and has a high likelihood of leading to destructive changes if not treated sufficiently.

The prevalence of PsA was underestimated in the past. Although no large-scale epidemiological studies have been performed, the prevalence was thought to be in the range of 5–8% of all patients with psoriasis of the skin. A major problem in determining the exact prevalence of PsA is the absence of a widely accepted definition. Over the years, different classification systems have been proposed with uncertainty about the best predictive system for PsA. Recently, a classification system with a higher specificity has been proposed by the CASPAR study group that is supposed to be easy to use, especially in survey studies, and might result in better reporting of PsA.

Up to now, numerous studies have tried to address the prevalence of PsA (table 1), leading to a wide range of prevalence rates. In a nationwide study in Germany, in which patients were first seen by a dermatologist and later referred to a rheumatologist when signs of arthritis were present, the estimated prevalence was 20.6%, which may be a better estimate of the true prevalence of PsA than the previous 5–8% [2].

Psoriasis and Crohn's Disease

Previous studies have provided evidence that patients suffering from at least one IMID are at a higher risk of another IMID [3]. Common immune-mediated disorders with a strong inflammatory component that are of primary interest include asthma, psoriasis,

Table 1. Prevalence of PsA in psoriasis patients

Reference	Year	Prevalence, %	Comments
Salvarani et al. [45]	1995	36	
Scarpa et al. [46]	1984	34.4	
Zachariae [47]	2003	30	
Alenius et al. [48]	2002	39	with enthesitis and undifferentiated spondylarthritides
Resch et al. [2]	2009	20.6	
Ferrandiz et al. [49]	2002	17.3	
Zanolli and Wikle [50]	1992	17	
Jajic and el Assadi [51]	2003	15.3	
Bell et al. [52]	1991	12.9	
Gelfand et al. [53]	2005	11	
Pavlica et al. [54]	2005	9.3	
Gisondi et al. [55]	2005	7.7	
Biondi et al. [56]	1994	1	juvenile PsA

type 1 diabetes, rheumatoid arthritis, multiple sclerosis, systemic lupus erythematosus, vitiligo, autoimmune thyroiditis and chronic glomerulonephritis. In a recent study evaluating data from 12,601 patients with inflammatory bowel disease (IBD), other IMID occurred at a greater frequency in IBD patients than in the general population. Asthma (odds ratio:1.5, 95% CI: 1.4–1.6), psoriasis (odds ratio: 1.7, 95% CI: 1.5–2.0), rheumatoid arthritis (odds ratio:1.9, 95% CI: 1.5–2.3) and multiple sclerosis (odds ratio:2.3, 95% CI: 1.6–3.3) were shown to have a higher prevalence as compared to a matched control group [4]. Smaller studies have already shown an increased prevalence of psoriasis and a familiar background of psoriasis in Crohn's disease as well as in ulcerative colitis. A possible genetic link has been described in recent years: non-MHC (major histocompatibility complex) psoriasis susceptibility loci tend to overlap with disease regions for other inflammatory disorders such as IBD [5]. It has for example been shown that Crohn's-disease-associated sequence variants in the interleukin 23 receptor (IL-23R) and interleukin 12 (IL-12B) genes lead to an increased risk of psoriasis [6–8]. The IL-12 and IL-23 pathways are of importance in Crohn's disease as well as in psoriasis. IL-12 mainly induces differentiation of CD4 naïve T cells to T helper 1 cells (TH1) and activates natural killer cells, which leads to a production of type 1 cytokines such as interferon-γ, IL-2 and tumor necrosis factor-α (TNFα). The dominant role of IL-23 may be the stimulation of a special subset of recently identified Th17 cells to produce IL-17, TNFα and IL-6, and to develop into a Th17 phenotype.

For Crohn's disease, the main focus now is on IL-23 as it was shown that antibodies against the p19 subunit specific for IL-23 suppress chronic intestinal inflammation in an IBD model [9]. The initial evidence from clinical trials demonstrates the therapeutic efficacy of an antibody to the p40 subunit of IL-12 and IL-23 in Crohn's disease and psoriasis, highlighting the pathophysiological importance of these cytokines [10–13].

Other genetic similarities between Crohn's disease and psoriasis are found in the HLA antigen region on chromosome 6p. Psoriasis susceptibility region 1 is located at 6p21 and the IBD susceptibility region 3 is also located at 6p. TNFα has proven to be of major importance for both diseases as it is found in increased levels in disease lesions and TNFα inhibitors are highly efficacious in both indications. The TNFα gene neighbors both disease susceptibility regions located at 6p21.3, and recent genetic analyses have linked polymorphisms of TNFα and its promotor region to Crohn's disease, psoriasis and psoriasis arthritis [14], although the exact positions of the single nucleotide polymorphisms found in these diseases differ. Several studies have shown functional polymorphisms in the –238 and –308 sites of the TNFα promotor region in psoriasis and psoriasis arthritis [14, 15], whereas the –308 site could not be associated with Crohn's disease [16]. Other TNFα promoter regions such as –1031, –863 and –857 have, at least in some studies, shown an association with Crohn's disease, although the data is still inconclusive [16].

Psoriasis and the Risk of Neoplasia

An increased incidence of malignancies in patients with psoriasis has been shown in several studies. This association of malignancies has been described as being caused by either psoriasis itself or certain systemic treatments of the disease. In most studies, increases in squamous cell skin carcinoma, non-Hodgkin and Hodgkin lymphoma, cutaneous T cell lymphoma and laryngeal cancer were present, although not all studies found an increased risk of associated malignancies in patients with psoriasis. In particular, the increased risk of head and neck malignancies (such as larynx, pharynx, esophagus and oral cavity cancers) may be related to aberrant alcohol and smoking habits of psoriasis patients. Besides these exogenous risk factors, the immunological nature of psoriasis may contribute to a pathophysiological association of the disease and an increase in lymphoma risk as this has been demonstrated in other TH1-associated diseases, such as rheumatoid arthritis. Furthermore, treatment of psoriasis with cyclosporine and methotrexate has been associated with the development of lymphoma. Numerous studies have tried to clarify the association of lymphoma and psoriasis. In a large population-based cohort study, 153,197 patients with psoriasis were compared to 765,950 corresponding subjects without psoriasis. In this study, an association between Hodgkin's disease and cutaneous T cell lymphoma was shown. The authors concluded that psoriasis patients are at a higher risk of developing lymphoproliferative diseases, but, as lymphoma is a rare disease and the magnitude of association is modest, the absolute risk attributable to psoriasis is low [17].

In a prospective long-term cohort study on severe psoriasis patients treated with cyclosporine, a standardized incidence ratio for malignancy of 2.1 was found compared to the general population, in which the higher incidence of malignancies was attributed to a 6-fold higher incidence of mainly squamous cell skin carcinoma. In particular, the duration of cyclosporine treatment or exposure to PUVA, methotrexate or immunosuppressants showed a significant effect on the incidence of non-melanoma skin cancers [18]. A similar result was published for a Finnish cohort study with 5,687 hospitalized psoriasis patients. The overall cancer incidence ratio was increased with a standardized incidence ratio of 1.3. The highest relative risks were estimated for Hodgkin's disease, squamous cell skin carcinoma, non-Hodgkin's lymphoma and laryngeal cancer. For squamous cell skin carcinoma, an association of oral PUVA therapy and retinoids was shown to have a relative risk of 6.5, whereas no association of treatments with non-Hodgkin's lymphoma was assessed [19].

A close follow-up of incidence rates of malignancies in psoriasis is recommended as new therapies selectively target specific components of the immune system and concern has been raised about whether these therapies may also contribute to the development of neoplasias. Prospective long-term follow-up studies could best help to elucidate this unsolved question.

Psoriasis and Metabolic Syndrome

An increasingly important association of psoriasis is with metabolic syndrome. Already in one of the first studies reporting comorbidities with psoriasis, hypertension, diabetes mellitus and dyslipoproteinemia were described, together with the fact that the majority of patients were obese [20].

There have been different classification systems for the metabolic syndrome over the years. The most widely used definitions include those of the World Health Organization, the US National Cholesterol Educational Program and the International Diabetes Federation. In all definitions, criteria for central obesity, raised triglyceride levels, reduced high-density lipoprotein cholesterol levels, insulin resistance and hypertension are involved, but do differ slightly and may influence the comparability of epidemiological studies. There have been data published on disease concomitance in psoriasis that revealed higher prevalence rates of diseases related to metabolic syndrome. Table 2 gives an overview of the recent literature and prevalence rates. Sommer et al. [21], Gisondi et al. [22] and Cohen et al. [23] were the only authors to calculate odds ratios for metabolic syndrome itself. The first study compared 581 adult patients hospitalized for plaque-type psoriasis with a hospital-based control group of 1,044 patients treated surgically for localized stage I melanoma. They found a higher prevalence of metabolic syndrome in psoriasis patients, with an odds ratio of 5.92 [21]. Gisondi et al. [22] performed a hospital-based case-control study on 338 adult patients with chronic plaque-type psoriasis and 334 patients with skin diseases

Table 2. Metabolic syndrome and associated diseases

	Diabetes mellitus		Hypertension		Dyslipidemia		Obesity		Metabolic syndrome	
	odds ratio	p value	odds ratio	p value	odds ratio	p value	odds ratio	p value	odds ratio	p value
Sommer et al. [21], 2006	2.48	<0.0001	3.27	<0.0001	2.09	<0.01	2.3[1]	<0.0001	5.29	<0.0001
Gisondi et al. [22], 2007	n.a.	n.s.[2]	n.a.	n.s.	n.a.	<0.001[3]	n.a.	<0.0001[4]	1.65	0.005
Henseler and Christophers [20], 1995	1.47	<0.05	1.9	<0.01	n.a.	n.a.	2.05	<0.05	n.a.	n.a.
Lindegård [57], 1986	n.a.	<0.001[5]	n.a.	<0.001	n.a.	n.a.	n.a.	0.005[5]	n.a.	n.a.
Mallbris et al. [58], 2006	n.a.	n.a.	n.a.	n.a.	1.15	< 0.001	n.a.	n.a.	n.a.	n.a.
Pearce et al. [59], 2005	1.03	<0.001[6]	1.05	<0.001[6]	1.04	<0.001[6]	n.a.	n.a.	n.a.	n.a.
Neimann et al. [31], 2006	1.86	sig.	1.25	sig.	1.31	sig.	1.84[7]	sig.	n.a.	n.a.
Gelfand et al. [35], 2006	n.a.	<0.001	n.a.	<0.001	n.a.	<0.001	n.a.	<0.001[8]	n.a.	n.a.
Cohen et al. [60], 2007	1.5	<0.001	1.3	<0.01	1.2	<0.05	1.3	<0.05	n.a.	n.a.
Cohen et al. [23], 2008	1.2		1.3		n.a.	n.a.	1.7		1.3	

n.s. = Not significant; n.a. = not applicable; sig. = significant.
[1] Logistic regression analysis.
[2] Fasting plasma glucose.
[3] Triglyceridemia.
[4] Body mass index.
[5] Only in females.
[6] Anti-gliadin antibodies as a continuous 1-year variable.
[7] Body mass index >30.
[8] Significantly higher body mass index.

other than psoriasis, and described a higher prevalence of psoriasis in patients after the age of 40 years with an odds ratio of 1.65 that was directly correlated to psoriasis duration [22]. The largest study (analyzing data from 16,851 patients with psoriasis and 48,681 control subjects), by Cohen et al. [23], used data from a national health service database. Even in this analysis involving large patient numbers, a higher prevalence of metabolic syndrome in patients with psoriasis was shown with an odds ratio of 1.3. The importance of this syndrome lies in its ability to predispose sufferers to CVD. It has been shown in cohort studies, such as the Framingham Offspring Study, that the presence of the metabolic syndrome is associated with an increased risk of CVD and type 2 diabetes mellitus in both sexes [24]. Furthermore, the total mortality rate was shown to be significantly higher in patients with, rather than without, metabolic syndrome. Several other studies on psoriasis have focused on single symptoms as part of metabolic syndrome. An impairment in lipid metabolism was shown by different groups. An unfavorable increase in the lipid profile was observed in association with the severity of psoriasis, with severely affected patients being at greater risk. All these findings lead to an increased risk of developing CVD. However, to estimate the overall CVD risk, all major cardiovascular risk factors have to be considered. This includes smoking status and body mass index (BMI).

Psoriasis and 'Lifestyle Factors'

Smoking, alcohol consumption and obesity are often referred to as 'lifestyle factors'. This term belittles the importance of these factors in association to psoriasis. As obesity is a separate disease with major impacts on the general health status of patients and a direct influence on other diseases such as diabetes, dyslipoproteinemia and CVD, it should not be subsumed under the term 'lifestyle factors'.

Psoriasis and Consumption of Nicotine and Alcohol

Smoking, in particular, has been correlated with psoriasis in numerous studies, and was even associated with the clinical severity in a study evaluating 818 adult hospitalized psoriasis patients [25]. The strongest link between smoking and skin manifestations was reported for pustular forms of psoriasis (i.e. plaque-type psoriasis associated with pustular lesions and generalized pustular psoriasis) with an odds ratio of 5.3 for current smokers in a study by Naldi et al. [26]. In some studies, smoking appeared to be a factor in the onset of the disease. In a cross-sectional study from the Utah Psoriasis Initiative, 78% of the patients reported that they began smoking before the onset of psoriasis [27]. Data from the literature suggest some gender differences in smoking habits. In 550 psoriasis patients from an Italian case-control study, psoriasis was more prevalent in male ex-smokers but male current smokers had a lower prevalence of psoriasis than female current smokers. The effect of cigarette-years on psoriasis severity was also shown to be stronger in women.

Higgins [28] concluded that smoking is a more prominent trigger factor for psoriasis in women than in men.

The available evidence on alcohol intake and psoriasis is less conclusive. Some earlier studies were not able to show an association of drinking habits and psoriasis, whereas other studies demonstrated an association both in men and in women. It was proposed that the earlier studies failed to show a correlation with the disease as they did not control for confounding factors such as tobacco use. When controlling for such factors, study results often demonstrated a significant correlation between alcohol use and psoriasis. Very recently, an association between weekly alcohol consumption and the severity of psoriasis has been observed in psoriasis patients [29].

Psoriasis and Obesity

Obesity is an increasing problem in western civilizations, accounting for up to 16% of the global burden of disease and 2–7% of the total health care expenditure [30]. Numerous studies have substantiated an even higher prevalence of obesity among psoriasis patients as compared to the general population. A correlation between the severity of psoriasis and the prevalence of obesity was described by Neimann et al. [31]. There is an ongoing controversial discussion on whether obesity precedes psoriasis or vice versa. The first indication that obesity may follow the onset of psoriasis was given by Herron et al. [27], who used a retrospective self-reported body image assessment tool.

Obesity itself, and especially visceral obesity, is a risk factor for coronary heart disease. Intra-abdominal fat is an endocrine organ producing multiple adipokines that play a role in insulin sensitivity, lipid metabolism and inflammation, which are linked to CVD [32]. Recent data indicate that central abdominal white adipose tissue is infiltrated by macrophages, which may be a major source of locally produced proinflammatory cytokines, such as IL-6 and TNFα, that lead to measurable elevated serum levels in obese patients. Adipokines such as adiponectin show insulin-sensitizing effects, and are supposed to protect against arteriosclerosis by counteracting with TNFα. Circulating levels of leptin are strongly associated with fat mass in obesity, and can lead to an increased inflammatory response. The main function of leptin seems to be the control of energy fat stores and regulating appetite and body weight in humans. The energy balance is negatively influenced by leptin in an abundant energy status by reducing appetite and increasing energy expenditure. Patients with leptin deficiency are extremely obese; even so, in obese patients leptin levels are increased without effecting the patient's general food intake, and the treatment of obese patients with exogenous leptin substitution has no effect. This led to the concept of leptin resistance in obesity, similar to insulin resistance in type 2 diabetes. In obesity, insulin resistance has been linked to leptin resistance and decreased plasma adiponectin. In a study analyzing data from 39 patients with moderate-to-severe plaque-type psoriasis, a correlation between insulin secretion as well as resistin levels and psoriasis severity has been shown [33], supporting a link between a chronic state of inflammation in obesity and chronic systemic inflammation in psoriasis. Taken together, these recent data give clear evidence that an obese state contributes to a proinflammatory condition and probably enhances inflammation in psoriasis and related comorbidities.

Recently published data on a prospective study of 78,626 women over a 14-year period examining the relationship between BMI, weight change, waist circumference, hip circumference and waist-to-hip ratio proved the hypothesis that obesity is a risk factor for developing psoriasis. The risk of incident psoriasis was positively correlated with increasing BMI [34]. With this knowledge about obesity leading to a proinflammatory state and being a risk factor for developing psoriasis, the question appears of whether or not weight loss could lead to less inflammation and improve the clinical outcome of psoriasis.

Psoriasis and CVD

As discussed, there are numerous risk factors for CVD, such as metabolic syndrome and other classic CVD risk factors that are associated with psoriasis. Most of the studies in the literature on CVD and risk factors are limited by a selected patient cohort, such as hospitalized patients with severe psoriasis. Furthermore, many studies did not perform statistic multivariate analyses to determine independent CVD risk factors for psoriasis. Neimann and et al. [31] recently conducted a population-based study, and showed an independent association of severe psoriasis with diabetes, smoking and increased BMI. Thus, psoriasis patients are at a high risk of developing CVD. Indeed, several studies demonstrated an increased risk of occlusive vascular disease, myocardial infarction (MI) and coronary artery calcification. In a representative population-based cohort analyzed to determine the risk of MI in psoriasis patients, including 130,976 psoriasis patients and 556,995 corresponding control subjects, an increased relative risk for MI (especially in younger men) was shown. This higher risk persisted when controlled for the major risk factors for MI, suggesting that psoriasis is an independent risk factor [35]. To assess the degree of coronary artery calcification in patients with an at least 10 years' history of psoriasis and no history of CVD, a recent study performed spiral computed tomography in 32 patients and matched controls. A significantly increased prevalence of coronary artery calcification in the psoriasis patient cohort could be shown, suggesting a potential effect of a systemic inflammatory processes in psoriasis on the coronary arteries [36]. This data is in accordance with other inflammatory diseases such as rheumatoid arthritis, which is also associated with an increased risk of CVD and MI. Interestingly, the situation in PsA is very similar to psoriasis. It seems possible that psoriasis is a disease associated with atherosclerosis, in which chronic and systemic inflammation play a key role in the pathogenesis. A higher prevalence of CVD and their risk factors have been demonstrated by epidemiological studies. A recent study evaluating carotid artery intima-media thickness by high-resolution ultrasound in 59 patients with PsA and without any other cardiovascular risk factors found a significantly increased prevalence of carotid artery intima-media thickness compared to matched controls [37].

Endothelial Dysfunction

The endothelium is most important in vascular structure, vascular tone and inflammatory processes; thus, representing the earliest affected structure in atherosclerotic disease and its worst complications such as MI and stroke. Endothelial dysfunction (ED) promotes arterial inflammation, and chronic inflammation promotes ED. Adhesive molecules and cytokines play a pivotal role in the inflamed atherosclerotic vascular wall [38]. In early atherosclerosis, it is mostly adhesive molecules that mediate cell adhesion between platelets, leukocytes and the vascular wall. Cytokine activation is secondary, and leads to an imbalance between pro- and anti-inflammatory actions. ED can be caused by all common cardiovascular risk factors; thus, linking ED to diseases such as dyslipidemia, diabetes, hypertension, as well as smoking and obesity. In many studies, it was shown that the degree of ED was related to future clinical cardiovascular events, and its assessment was discussed as a potential marker for patients at risk of CVD.

In a recent study of 50 patients with PsA without any cardiovascular risk factor or a history of cardiovascular or cerebrovascular events, the presence of ED by measuring flow-mediated endothelial-dependent vasodilatation was shown [39]. This study supports the existence of impaired endothelial function in a patient cohort suffering from a chronic inflammatory disease without any clinical sign of CVD. For rheumatoid arthritis as another chronic inflammatory disease, the importance of atherosclerosis as a leading factor in reduced life expectancy is widely acknowledged. The underlying inflammatory state has been described as the most important mechanism for ED and early atherosclerosis in rheumatoid arthritis [40]. In general, the inflammatory process is seen as an important factor underlying the pathogenesis of atherosclerosis at every step.

In diabetes mellitus, ED is universal and represents an early sign of diabetic vasculopathy; it is an independent predictor of cardiovascular risk. Presumably, the uncoupling of endothelial nitric oxide synthase is a major factor in the pathogenetic mechanism of ED in type 2 diabetes mellitus. Interestingly, the main factors that cause the suggested biochemical disturbances are dyslipoproteinemia, oxidative stress and inflammation.

Hypertension increases shear stress on the endothelium, and may result in endothelial cell activation or even damage. Adipose tissue in obesity produces inflammatory markers that can stimulate the expression of cellular adhesion molecules and support the development of ED. Taken together, nearly all diseases of metabolic syndrome such as hypertension, diabetes mellitus, dyslipidemia and obesity are correlated to ED.

To date, no study has been available that investigated ED in patients with plaque-type psoriasis, but there is a great chance that it will be found in this patient group as most of the diseases leading to ED and an inflammatory state are present in psoriasis.

Role of Comedication

As already discussed, comorbidities are more frequently found in psoriasis patients as compared to the general population, and almost all of these comorbidities require systemic treatment. It is well known that some drugs or drug classes have the potential to trigger psoriasis, which has been show in particular for the groups of β-blockers and antimalarials in the past. Recent data provide accumulating evidence that the risk of triggering psoriasis is also present with ACE inhibitors [41]. ACE inhibitors and ß-blockers are frequently used in the treatment of hypertension, which is part of metabolic syndrome and one of the most frequently found comorbidities in psoriasis. In a recent nationwide survey in Germany, which assessed the state of comedications used on psoriasis patients hospitalized for treatment of a severe form of the disease (mean Psoriasis Area and Severity Index score: 26), ACE inhibitors were used by 12.5% and β-blockers by 7.9% of all patients. Compared to the general population, the use of β-blockers in the treatment of hypertension was lower, but this was partly compensated by the more frequent use of ACE inhibitors in the patients with psoriasis [42].

Another underestimated risk from a different perspective is the influence of systemic antipsoriatic treatment on psoriatic comorbidities. Frequently found comorbidities could be aggravated by antipsoriatic drugs. Therapy with the retinoid acitretin has a good chance of increasing serum triglycerides and cholesterol, negatively influencing the pre-existing dyslipoproteinemia linked to metabolic syndrome. Ciclosporin, an effective compound in the treatment of psoriasis, could lead to deterioration or first onset of hypertension, and may also increase serum lipids and thus the risk of ED and CVD. If iatrogenic hypertension needs to be treated for medical reasons with ACE inhibitors or ß-blockers, this again could negatively influence the patients' skin symptoms. The most frequently used antipsoriatic drug worldwide, methotrexate, has to be used with caution in patients with diabetes, particularly insulin-dependent diabetes and excessive alcohol intake. Thus, comorbidities not only reduce therapeutic options, but can also be aggravated by antipsoriatic treatment if not carefully considered before treatment initiation.

In the previously mentioned German comedication survey, the overall intake of comedication was significant: 60.1% of all severely affected patients with psoriasis were regularly receiving systemic medication, and 30% took 3 or more different drugs [42]. For some antipsoriatic medications, such as methotrexate and ciclosporin, there is a high risk of drug interactions, whereas retinoids show a lower risk, and biologics or fumaric acid esters have no known risk of interaction, which has to be considered when treating these patients. Comedications can also influence antipsoriatic UV treatment as photosensitivity can be caused by different agents, such as thiazide diuretics and tetracyclines. Diuretics, in particular, are frequently used in concomitant hypertension. In the German comedication survey, 17% of all severely affected patients with psoriasis had been treated with diuretics [42].

Relevance of Comorbidities

The understanding of psoriasis being a systemic inflammatory condition rather than a single organ disease is increasingly accepted in the medical community. Current data provide increasing evidence that psoriasis is associated with numerous comorbidities. Besides PsA, the association with diseases such as metabolic syndrome is especially prominent and contributes to the increased risk of CVD and its medical consequences, particularly in severely affected psoriasis patients. Heavy smoking and alcohol consumption are further risk factors that have been shown to contribute to an increased risk of dying among moderate to severe affected psoriasis patients.

A common feature linking most of the recognized comorbidities and psoriasis is the inflammatory state of these diseases, which may at least in part explain these associations. Obesity, for example, contributes to an underlying proinflammatory state by producing cytokines such as TNFα and IL-6. TNFα itself is an important mediator of insulin resistance, and can lead to the development of diabetes. In PsA and Crohn's disease, these cytokines are as important as in psoriasis – indirectly proven by the efficacy of anti-TNFα therapy in all of these diseases.

Many comorbidities of psoriasis are risk factors for CVD and MI. However, psoriasis itself has now been identified as being independently associated with CVD.

The attention of the dermatologist and other physicians taking care of patients with psoriasis should focus on early intervention to prevent the development of CVD, atherosclerosis and its consequences. Supposing that the systemic inflammatory state of psoriasis is of major importance, antipsoriatic treatment could reduce the incidence of vascular diseases. In a retrospective cohort study of 7,615 psoriasis patients receiving methotrexate therapy, a significantly reduced risk of vascular diseases, particularly in low- to moderate-dose regimes in combination with folic acid supplementation, was observed [43]. In other IMID, such as rheumatoid arthritis which is also associated with increased mortality and morbidity due to atherosclerosis, a beneficial effect of anti-TNFα therapy has been shown. In particular, patients that responded to anti-TNFα therapy showed a markedly reduced risk of MI. Regarding psoriasis, it may be assumed that anti-TNFα therapy or systemic treatment with other immunomodulating drugs will provide the same beneficial protective effect.

A stronger focus on comorbidities should improve the management of patients with psoriasis through better interdisciplinary cooperation involving multiple medical disciplines besides dermatology. In addition, health care providers must acknowledge that psoriasis is not only a primarily benign disease of the skin, but represents a complex systemic disorder with various possible complications and associated problems.

Role of Dermatologists in the Management of Patients with Psoriasis

The dermatologist is usually the health care specialist that is first and most often consulted by patients with psoriasis, and often becomes the manager and primary care keeper of patients' preventive health care needs. In a survey analyzing data from 74 psoriasis patients seen for the first time in our own psoriasis center, 70.3% of the patients wished to be seen regularly and 39.1% wished to always be seen by a dermatologist. As severe psoriasis needs to be considered as a systemic disease, it may become the responsibility of the dermatologist to recognize early signs of underlying comorbidities and to refer the patient to other specialists (e.g. rheumatologists, cardiologists, psychiatrists or diabetologists) to ensure an interdisciplinary treatment approach to these patients.

The National Psoriasis Foundation has addressed this central role of the dermatologists, and proposed possible screening recommendations for comorbidities. Recommendations to assess the general cardiovascular risk follow the American Heart Association guidelines from 2002. Risk factor screening should start at the age of 20 years, and should include blood pressure measurements, evaluation of BMI, waist circumference and pulse rate, at least every 2 years from the age of 40 years, as well as monitoring of cholesterol and fasting blood glucose every 5 years. Patients with risk factors for CVD may need to be monitored more closely. For patients already suffering from metabolic syndrome, the American Heart Association guidelines recommend a weight loss to achieve a BMI of less than 25, physical activity for 30 min most days of the week and healthy eating habits. Smoking cessation and moderating alcohol intake may also show beneficial effects on CVD and psoriasis [44].

Besides these screening recommendations for metabolic syndrome and cardiovascular risk factors, other well-established comorbidities such as PsA have to be kept in mind. All patients with psoriasis should routinely be screened for early signs of PsA, as the majority of patients affected are first seen by a dermatologist. Early detection and intervention are the only possibilities to prevent long-term joint damage in PsA patients. Therefore, an interdisciplinary approach with rheumatologists is extremely important to manage psoriasis patients with concomitant PsA sufficiently.

Conclusion

Regardless of the high importance of comorbidities, the aim of a dermatologist treating patients with psoriasis should still be the sufficient treatment of skin symptoms and the resulting impairment in patients' quality of life. However, severe psoriasis is a systemic disease with numerous potential comorbidities, and dermatologists are becoming managers of an interdisciplinary treatment approach for this subgroup of patients. The patients should be routinely screened for possible signs of concomitant diseases for early detection. Sufficient antipsoriatic treatment may not only improve patients' skin symptoms, but also their comorbidities, leading to long-term control of psoriasis and possibly to the prevention of long-term complications.

References

1 Khan MA: Update on spondyloarthropathies. Ann Intern Med 2002;136:896–907.

2 Reich K, Krüger K, Mössner R, Augustin M: Epidemiology and clinical pattern of psoriatic arthritis in Germany: a prospective interdisciplinary epidemiological study of 1,511 patients with plaque-type psoriasis. Br J Dermatol 2009. E-pub ahead of print.

3 Robinson D Jr, Hackett M, Wong J, Kimball AB, Cohen R, Bala M: Co-occurrence and comorbidities in patients with immune-mediated inflammatory disorders: an exploration using US healthcare claims data, 2001–2002. Curr Med Res Opin 2006;22:989–1000.

4 Weng X, Liu L, Barcellos LF, Allison JE, Herrinton LJ: Clustering of inflammatory bowel disease with immune mediated diseases among members of a Northern California-managed care organization. Am J Gastroenterol 2007;102:1429–1435.

5 Wolf N, Quaranta M, Prescott N, Allen M, Smith R, Burden AD, et al: Psoriasis is associated with pleiotropic susceptibility loci identified in type II diabetes and Crohn's disease. J Med Genet 2008;45: 114–116.

6 Duerr RH, Taylor KD, Brant SR, Rioux JD, Silverberg MS, Daly MJ, et al: A genome-wide association study identifies IL23R as an inflammatory bowel disease gene. Science 2006;314:1461–1463.

7 Capon F, Di Meglio P, Szaub J, Prescott NJ, Dunster C, Baumber L, et al: Sequence variants in the genes for the interleukin-23 receptor (IL23R) and its ligand (IL12B) confer protection against psoriasis. Hum Genet 2007;122:201–206.

8 Cargill M, Schrodi SJ, Chang M, Garcia VE, Brandon R, Callis KP, et al: A large-scale genetic association study confirms IL12B and leads to the identification of IL23R as psoriasis-risk genes. Am J Hum Genet 2007;80:273–290.

9 Neurath MF: IL-23: a master regulator in Crohn disease. Nat Med 2007;13:26–28.

10 Krueger GG, Langley RG, Leonardi C, Yeilding N, Guzzo C, Wang Y, et al: A human interleukin-12/23 monoclonal antibody for the treatment of psoriasis. N Engl J Med 2007;356:580–592.

11 Papp KA, Langley RG, Lebwohl M, Krueger GG, Szapary P, Yeilding N, et al: Efficacy and safety of ustekinumab, a human interleukin-12/23 monoclonal antibody, in patients with psoriasis: 52-week results from a randomised, double-blind, placebo-controlled trial (PHOENIX 2). Lancet 2008;371: 1675–1684.

12 Leonardi CL, Kimball AB, Papp KA, Yeilding N, Guzzo C, Wang Y, et al: Efficacy and safety of ustekinumab, a human interleukin-12/23 monoclonal antibody, in patients with psoriasis: 76-week results from a randomised, double-blind, placebo-controlled trial (PHOENIX 1). Lancet 2008;371:1665–1674.

13 Mannon PJ, Fuss IJ, Mayer L, Elson CO, Sandborn WJ, Present D, et al: Anti-interleukin-12 antibody for active Crohn's disease. N Engl J Med 2004;351: 2069–2079.

14 Reich K, Huffmeier U, Konig IR, Lascorz J, Lohmann J, Wendler J, et al: TNF polymorphisms in psoriasis: association of psoriatic arthritis with the promoter polymorphism TNF*-857 independent of the PSORS1 risk allele. Arthritis Rheum 2007;56:2056–2064.

15 Li C, Wang G, Gao Y, Liu L, Gao T: TNF-alpha gene promoter –238G>A and –308G>A polymorphisms alter risk of psoriasis vulgaris: a meta-analysis. J Invest Dermatol 2007;127:1886–1892.

16 Zipperlen K, Peddle L, Melay B, Hefferton D, Rahman P: Association of TNF-alpha polymorphisms in Crohn disease. Hum Immunol 2005;66: 56–59.

17 Gelfand JM, Shin DB, Neimann AL, Wang X, Margolis DJ, Troxel AB: The risk of lymphoma in patients with psoriasis. J Invest Dermatol 2006;126: 2194–2201.

18 Paul CF, Ho VC, McGeown C, Christophers E, Schmidtmann B, Guillaume JC, et al: Risk of malignancies in psoriasis patients treated with cyclosporine: a 5 y cohort study. J Invest Dermatol 2003; 120:211–216.

19 Hannuksela-Svahn A, Pukkala E, Laara E, Poikolainen K, Karvonen J: Psoriasis, its treatment, and cancer in a cohort of Finnish patients. J Invest Dermatol 2000;114:587–590.
20 Henseler T, Christophers E: Disease concomitance in psoriasis. J Am Acad Dermatol 1995;32:982–986.
21 Sommer DM, Jenisch S, Suchan M, Christophers E, Weichenthal M: Increased prevalence of the metabolic syndrome in patients with moderate to severe psoriasis. Arch Dermatol Res 2006;298:321–328.
22 Gisondi P, Tessari G, Conti A, Piaserico S, Schianchi S, Peserico A, et al: Prevalence of metabolic syndrome in patients with psoriasis: a hospital-based case-control study. Br J Dermatol 2007;157:68–73.
23 Cohen AD, Sherf M, Vidavsky L, Vardy DA, Shapiro J, Meyerovitch J: Association between psoriasis and the metabolic syndrome: a cross-sectional study. Dermatology 2008;216:152–155.
24 Wilson PW, D'Agostino RB, Parise H, Sullivan L, Meigs JB: Metabolic syndrome as a precursor of cardiovascular disease and type 2 diabetes mellitus. Circulation 2005;112:3066–3072.
25 Fortes C, Mastroeni S, Leffondre K, Sampogna F, Melchi F, Mazzotti E, et al: Relationship between smoking and the clinical severity of psoriasis. Arch Dermatol 2005;141:1580–1584.
26 Naldi L, Chatenoud L, Linder D, Belloni FA, Peserico A, Virgili AR, et al: Cigarette smoking, body mass index, and stressful life events as risk factors for psoriasis: results from an Italian case-control study. J Invest Dermatol 2005;125:61–67.
27 Herron MD, Hinckley M, Hoffman MS, Papenfuss J, Hansen CB, Callis KP, et al: Impact of obesity and smoking on psoriasis presentation and management. Arch Dermatol 2005;141:1527–1534.
28 Higgins E: Alcohol, smoking and psoriasis. Clin Exp Dermatol 2000;25:107–110.
29 Kirby B, Richards HL, Mason DL, Fortune DG, Main CJ, Griffiths CE: Alcohol consumption and psychological distress in patients with psoriasis. Br J Dermatol 2008;158:138–140.
30 Hossain P, Kawar B, El Nahas M: Obesity and diabetes in the developing world – a growing challenge. N Engl J Med 2007;356:213–215.
31 Neimann AL, Shin DB, Wang X, Margolis DJ, Troxel AB, Gelfand JM: Prevalence of cardiovascular risk factors in patients with psoriasis. J Am Acad Dermatol 2006;55:829–835.
32 Ronti T, Lupattelli G, Mannarino E: The endocrine function of adipose tissue: an update. Clin Endocrinol (Oxf) 2006;64:355–365.
33 Boehncke S, Thaci D, Beschmann H, Ludwig RJ, Ackermann H, Badenhoop K, et al: Psoriasis patients show signs of insulin resistance. Br J Dermatol 2007;157:1249–1251.
34 Setty AR, Curhan G, Choi HK: Obesity, waist circumference, weight change, and the risk of psoriasis in women: Nurses' Health Study II. Arch Intern Med 2007;167:1670–1675.
35 Gelfand JM, Neimann AL, Shin DB, Wang X, Margolis DJ, Troxel AB: Risk of myocardial infarction in patients with psoriasis. JAMA 2006;296:1735–1741.
36 Ludwig RJ, Herzog C, Rostock A, Ochsendorf FR, Zollner TM, Thaci D, et al: Psoriasis: a possible risk factor for development of coronary artery calcification. Br J Dermatol 2007;156:271–276.
37 Gonzalez-Juanatey C, Llorca J, Amigo-Diaz E, Dierssen T, Martin J, Gonzalez-Gay MA: High prevalence of subclinical atherosclerosis in psoriatic arthritis patients without clinically evident cardiovascular disease or classic atherosclerosis risk factors. Arthritis Rheum 2007;57:1074–1080.
38 Giannotti G, Landmesser U: Endothelial dysfunction as an early sign of atherosclerosis. Herz 2007;32:568–572.
39 Gonzalez-Juanatey C, Llorca J, Miranda-Filloy JA, Amigo-Diaz E, Testa A, Garcia-Porrua C, et al: Endothelial dysfunction in psoriatic arthritis patients without clinically evident cardiovascular disease or classic atherosclerosis risk factors. Arthritis Rheum 2007;57:287–293.
40 Del Rincón I, Williams K, Stern MP, Freeman GL, O'Leary DH, Escalante A: Association between carotid atherosclerosis and markers of inflammation in rheumatoid arthritis patients and healthy subjects. Arthritis Rheum 2003;48:1833–1840.
41 Cohen AD, Bonneh DY, Reuveni H, Vardy DA, Naggan L, Halevy S: Drug exposure and psoriasis vulgaris: case-control and case-crossover studies. Acta Derm Venereol 2005;85:299–303.
42 Gerdes S, Zahl VA, Knopf H, Weichenthal M, Mrowietz U: Comedication related to comorbidities: a study in 1,203 hospitalized patients with severe psoriasis. Br J Dermatol 2008;159:1116–1123.
43 Prodanovich S, Ma F, Taylor JR, Pezon C, Fasihi T, Kirsner RS: Methotrexate reduces incidence of vascular diseases in veterans with psoriasis or rheumatoid arthritis. J Am Acad Dermatol 2005;52:262–267.
44 Kimball AB, Gladman D, Gelfand JM, Gordon K, Horn EJ, Korman NJ, et al: National Psoriasis Foundation clinical consensus on psoriasis comorbidities and recommendations for screening. J Am Acad Dermatol 2008;58:1031–1042.
45 Salvarani C, Lo SG, Macchioni P, Cremonesi T, Rossi F, Mantovani W, et al: Prevalence of psoriatic arthritis in Italian psoriatic patients. J Rheumatol 1995;22:1499–1503.

46 Scarpa R, Oriente P, Pucino A, Torella M, Vignone L, Riccio A, et al: Psoriatic arthritis in psoriatic patients. Br J Rheumatol 1984;23:246–250.

47 Zachariae H: Prevalence of joint disease in patients with psoriasis: implications for therapy. Am J Clin Dermatol 2003;4:441–447.

48 Alenius GM, Stenberg B, Stenlund H, Lundblad M, Dahlqvist SR: Inflammatory joint manifestations are prevalent in psoriasis: prevalence study of joint and axial involvement in psoriatic patients, and evaluation of a psoriatic and arthritic questionnaire. J Rheumatol 2002;29:2577–2582.

49 Ferrandiz C, Pujol RM, Garcia-Patos V, Bordas X, Smandia JA: Psoriasis of early and late onset: a clinical and epidemiologic study from Spain. J Am Acad Dermatol 2002;46:867–873.

50 Zanolli MD, Wikle JS: Joint complaints in psoriasis patients. Int J Dermatol 1992;31:488–491.

51 Jajic Z, el Assadi G: Prevalence of psoriatic arthritis in a population of patients with psoriasis (in Croatian). Acta Med Croatica 2003;57:323–326.

52 Bell LM, Sedlack R, Beard CM, Perry HO, Michet CJ, Kurland LT: Incidence of psoriasis in Rochester, Minn, 1980–1983. Arch Dermatol 1991;127:1184–1187.

53 Gelfand JM, Gladman DD, Mease PJ, Smith N, Margolis DJ, Nijsten T, et al: Epidemiology of psoriatic arthritis in the population of the United States. J Am Acad Dermatol 2005;53:573.

54 Pavlica L, Peric-Hajzler Z, Jovelic A, Sekler B, Damjanovic M: Psoriatic arthritis: a retrospective study of 162 patients. Vojnosanit Pregl 2005;62:613–620.

55 Gisondi P, Girolomoni G, Sampogna F, Tabolli S, Abeni D: Prevalence of psoriatic arthritis and joint complaints in a large population of Italian patients hospitalised for psoriasis. Eur J Dermatol 2005;15: 279–283.

56 Biondi OC, Scarpa R, Oriente P: Prevalence and clinical features of juvenile psoriatic arthritis in 425 psoriatic patients. Acta Derm Venereol Suppl (Stockh) 1994;186:109–110.

57 Lindegard B: Diseases associated with psoriasis in a general population of 159,200 middle-aged, urban, native Swedes. Dermatologica 1986;172:298–304.

58 Mallbris L, Granath F, Hamsten A, Stahle M: Psoriasis is associated with lipid abnormalities at the onset of skin disease. J Am Acad Dermatol 2006; 54:614–621.

59 Pearce DJ, Morrison AE, Higgins KB, Crane MM, Balkrishnan R, Fleischer AB Jr, et al: The comorbid state of psoriasis patients in a university dermatology practice. J Dermatolog Treat 2005;16:319–323.

60 Cohen AD, Gilutz H, Henkin Y, Zahger D, Shapiro J, Bonneh DY, et al: Psoriasis and the metabolic syndrome. Acta Derm Venereol 2007;87:506–509.

Sascha Gerdes, MD
Department of Dermatology, UKSH, Campus Kiel
Schittenhelmstrasse 7
DE–24105 Kiel (Germany)
Tel. +49 431 5971512, Fax +49 431 5971543, E-Mail sgerdes@dermatology.uni-kiel.de

Yawalkar N (ed): Management of Psoriasis.
Curr Probl Dermatol. Basel, Karger, 2009, vol 38, pp 37–58

Topical Treatment of Psoriasis

Qurat ul Ain Kamili · Alan Menter

Psoriasis Research Unit, Baylor Research Institute, Dallas, Tex., USA

Abstract

Topical therapy forms the cornerstone in the management of psoriasis. Of significant value as monotherapy in mild to moderate psoriasis, it is used predominantly as adjunctive therapy in moderate and severe forms of the disease. Over the past decade, topical treatment of psoriasis has evolved from the age-old applications of tar and dithranol to the more acceptable and efficacious options of topical corticosteroids, retinoids and vitamin D analogues, with the advent of a wide range of appropriately tailored vehicles and sophisticated delivery modes. To ensure therapeutic success, proper patient education about the disease, the treatment options, their specific application modality and adverse effects is essential. This will help alleviate the common problem of poor patient adherence, and inevitably result in more optimal clinical outcomes.

A wide variety of therapeutic options are available to treat psoriasis, including topical preparations, phototherapy, and systemic and biological agents. The approach to treatment must be individualized on the basis of disease parameters such as the nature, extent, severity and duration of disease, the anatomical sites involved, and the response to previous therapy. In addition, patient-specific parameters, such as age, sex, general health, quality of life issues and each individual's understanding about their disease, all need to be considered. Of utmost importance is the physician and staff's sympathetic approach, emotional support, reassurance and proper patient education about the disease and treatment options. All these factors play a pivotal role in the management of the disease.

Topical therapy remains the mainstay of therapy in the management of psoriasis for the majority of patients, being used predominantly for mild to moderate disease as monotherapy and as adjunctive therapy for recalcitrant lesions in patients with moderate to severe disease.

While the delivery of the active drug locally to the skin with little concern about systemic side effects may appear simple, topical therapy is often time-consuming, and thus requires education and adherence. It has been observed that physicians generally presume that their patients follow their instructions more closely than they actually do. Therefore, it is important to simplify topical therapy as far as possible and educate each and every patient on the nuances of this important modality of therapy for psoriasis.

Severity Assessment

The management of psoriasis requires the clinician to perform an accurate and reliable assessment of disease severity. Severity of psoriasis has traditionally been determined by the physical extent of the disease, psychosocial impairment in quality of life, and previous response to therapy. A globally accepted uniform scoring system is of utmost importance in the comparison of treatment results obtained in clinical trials so that the knowledge can be applied in clinical practice, as currently the majority of clinicians do not use the clinical trials' criteria in daily practice.

In simple terms, mild psoriasis has been defined as affecting less than 5% of the body surface area (BSA), with moderate disease affecting 5–10%, and severe disease greater than 10% [1].

While percent BSA involvement, in which the area of the patient's palm (outstretched hand including all 5 digits) represents about 1% of total BSA, is a convenient and quick tool to assess extent of involvement, it does not take into account individual features of erythema, induration and scaling, or impact on the quality of life; all of these are significant indicators of disease morbidity.

The Psoriasis Assessment and Severity Index (PASI) was developed for use in assessing the response to a retinoid in a clinical trial [2]. Although it was not initially intended to be the standard assessment tool, it became a popular research tool and has subsequently been used to assess clinical response in the majority of trials. The PASI is calculated using a formula measuring erythema, induration and scaling of an average lesion and its extent and anatomical site, resulting in a single score for psoriasis severity from 0 to 72. Despite its popular use, it is an insensitive measure of psoriasis of limited extent. Thus, patients with disabling psoriasis, e.g. palmoplantar psoriasis, may have low PASI scores. Also, it fails to take into account the impact of the patient's psoriasis on their quality of life. The majority of clinical trials consider a reduction in the PASI score from baseline of 75% (PASI 75) or more to be the benchmark endpoint in assessing response to therapy.

The Physician's Global Assessment (PGA; or Investigator's Global Assessment) provides an overall subjective evaluation of disease severity and summarizes the quality of the psoriatic plaques relative to the baseline assessment. A 7-point ordinal scale is used to assess global severity using categories from 'clear' to 'severe', scored as 0–6, respectively. The PGA is however interpreted differently by different investigators. Also, individual assessment of plaque morphology (such as erythema, induration and scaling), degree of BSA involvement and impact on quality of life is not taken into consideration.

The Lattice System PGA, formerly known as Lattice System Global Psoriasis Score, combines psoriatic plaque quality with extent of BSA involvement [3]. It is a PGA for quantifying psoriasis severity in an 8-step score, ranging from 'clear' to 'very severe'.

The Salford Psoriasis Index takes a holistic approach on physician's assessment, psychosocial disability and treatment resistance. It incorporates the extent of psoriasis based on PASI (S; on a scale of 0–10), psychosocial disability (P; on a visual analogue score of 0–10) and past severity based on historical information (I; cumulative score incorporating previous therapies and length of use).

Scoring systems like PASI and PGA fail to take into account the impact on quality of life and patient's perception of well-being. The National Psoriasis Foundation's psoriasis score takes into account the patient's and investigator's global assessment of severity, making it a useful alternate means of assessing clinical activity.

The Koo-Menter Psoriasis Index has been designed as a practical tool in clinical practice to identify patients who may be candidates for systemic therapy. It consists of both the patient's assessment and physician's evaluation of the disease using a 12-point scale to assess psoriasis-specific health-related quality of life.

The 'rule of tens' recently proposed by Finlay [4] is an easily remembered concept to help define severe psoriasis: BSA involvement of >10%, PASI score of >10 or Dermatology Life Quality Index (DLQI) >10. Patients fulfilling any of the 3 criteria are considered to have severe psoriasis for which active/systemic intervention is required.

Recently, the Copenhagen Psoriasis Severity Index [5] has been introduced, which assesses plaque characteristics at specific body sites. It is similar to PASI, with the advantage of being simpler and incorporating meaningful representation of different anatomical areas.

Although there are many tools available to study the extent of disease and response to therapy, their validity and reliability need to be adequately investigated. A global scoring system, including physical, quality of life, joint and patient satisfaction indices is currently in clinical trial and under development by the International Psoriasis Council.

Emollients

Emollient use in psoriasis has been present since time immemorial, representing an internationally accepted adjunctive therapeutic approach to the treatment of psoriasis. Emollients hydrate the stratum corneum and reduce dryness and itchiness of the skin. Petrolatum in emollients may lead to inhibition of arachidonic acid metabolism, while also improving barrier recovery in irritated skin.

Emollients can be used as ointments, creams, lotions, soap substitutes or bath oils.

While in common use, few comparative studies regarding the efficacy of emollients have been carried out. The addition of water in oil emollients to a topical corticosteroid regimen demonstrated efficacy, and was shown to have a steroid-sparing effect.

Adverse effects with the use of emollients, such as folliculitis are rare, with occasional sensitization noted. Greasier emollients, which are water-in-oil based, are considered more effective; however, these are cosmetically less acceptable to patients.

Salicylic Acid

Mechanism of Action

Salicylic acid is a topical keratolytic agent that softens the psoriatic plaque and reduces the pH of the stratum corneum, thereby increasing hydration of the skin.

It is generally combined with topical corticosteroids to enhance penetration, especially for the management of more hypertrophic plaques on the scalp, palms and soles. A randomized controlled double-blinded multicenter trial revealed that a combination of mometasone furoate and salicylic acid was significantly more effective than mometasone furoate alone [6]. The ability of salicylic acid to enhance corticosteroid efficacy was also demonstrated in a double-blind 3-week study, in which in a bilateral comparison study of 0.05% betamethasone dipropionate and 3% salicylic acid combination was compared to 0.025% budesonide [7]. Erythema and induration was reduced more significantly on the sites where the combination ointment was applied. Steroid/salicylic acid combinations are not currently available in the USA. A comparative study of tacrolimus and salicylic acid combination versus tacrolimus alone in patients with psoriasis also revealed improved efficacy with the addition of salicylic acid [8].

Adverse Effects

Salicylic acid has the potential to cause skin irritation, and prolonged use over large areas (>20%) can lead to systemic toxicity, especially in children, or adults with renal or hepatic impairments.

Salicylic acid also blocks UVB radiation, and therefore must not be applied prior to phototherapy; it may however be used after the exposure. It also inactivates calcipotriene; therefore, the 2 drugs should not be used concurrently.

Tar

Coal tar is a complex mixture of substances produced during carbonization and distillation of coal. It roughly comprises 48% hydrocarbons, 42% carbon and 10% water. However standardization is poor; therefore, clinical studies on tar may not be comparable.

Mechanism of Action

The exact mechanism of action of tar, although not well characterized, includes antiproliferative, antipruritic and antibacterial effects. It also has a photosensitizing action. The specific active ingredients responsible for its efficacy are still not known.

Tar is available in various forms, including ointments, creams, lotions, shampoos, soaps and a newly developed 'roll on' preparation, either alone or in combination with other agents such as salicylic acid. Crude coal tar can be refined with alcohol extraction to yield liquor carbonis detergens, which is commonly used in scalp preparations or elsewhere in the body including palms and soles (palmoplantar psoriasis). Crude tar/liquor carbonis detergens has been decolorized with lead acetate in an attempt to make it cosmetically more acceptable.

The Goeckerman [9] regimen, utilizing crude coal tar combined with ultraviolet (UV) light, was initially used in the inpatient setting in 1925. It consisted of applying 2–5% crude tar ointment combined with a tar bath and gradually increasing UVB irradiation. Different modifications have been tried for this regimen, including altering the concentration and timing of application in an attempt to make it more convenient for day care or outpatient therapy.

Despite its universal use, very few observational studies of tar have been carried out. In a double-blind randomized controlled trial, the efficacy of a 1% coal tar lotion (Exorex®) was compared with a 5% coal tar extract (Alphosyl®) in 324 patients with mild to moderate psoriasis [10]. It was concluded that patients treated with 1% coal tar lotion showed a better improvement in PASI and total sign scores than those treated with the conventional 5% extract.

Adverse Effects

Coal tar is inconvenient because of its unpleasant odor, staining of clothes and messiness (fig. 1). Irritant contact dermatitis, folliculitis, acneiform eruptions and photosensitivity reactions may also further limit its use. Although polycyclic hydrocarbons are known to be carcinogenic, there are no convincing data in humans showing an increased risk of cancers [11]. Tar is contraindicated in unstable psoriasis and on the face and flexures.

Dithranol

Dithranol, also known as anthralin, is 1,8-dihydroxy-9-anthrone.

Mechanism of Action

The induction of free radicals in the skin by dithranol results in antiproliferative effects and modulation of inflammation in psoriasis [12]. Recent studies have revealed that dithranol's mechanism of action is via a direct effect on mitochondria [12].

A mainstay of treatment for almost a century, its use has fallen steadily with the advent of more cosmetically acceptable therapies. It was initially used according to the regime of Ingram [13], which consisted of a daily tar bath and UV therapy, followed by a 24-hour application of dithranol paste containing salicylic acid (which prevents oxidative inactivation of dithranol). The concentration of the preparation is progressively increased from 0.05 up to 4%, depending on the degree of response and tolerance. Short contact application of high-dose dithranol for 30–60 min a day was shown to have a similar efficacy to a longer application time while being more convenient for patients [14].

Data studying efficacy of dithranol in comparison with other topical agents is flawed due to differences in drug concentrations, protocols and end points. Dithranol, tar and UVB/tar combinations appear to be roughly similar in efficacy.

Adverse Effects

The use of dithranol is limited by irritation and staining of the skin, nails, clothing and furniture. Application of trichloroethanolamine [15] as a wash-off solution following removal of dithranol can reduce the degree of irritation and staining, as does the short-contact regimen.

Newer formulations of dithranol have more favorable patient acceptability. Micanol®, in which dithranol is microencapsulated in crystalline monoglycerides, is hypothesized to deliver the active substance directly to the dermis; thereby, causing lower irritancy to the skin [16] (see 'New formulations' for recent additions).

Corticosteroids

Topical corticosteroid preparations remain the most widely prescribed topical treatment to treat psoriasis, especially in the USA. They are available in various strengths and formulations that enable the clinician to tailor the treatment according to the patient's requirements and preferences.

The Stoughton Cornell classification ranks the potency and clinical efficacy of topical corticosteroids on the basis of their ability to induce vasoconstriction [17]. In the UK, topical corticosteroids are classified into 4 groups; while in the USA, 7 classes are recognized. Clobetasol propionate (0.05%), available for over 3 decades, remains the most widely used potent topical corticosteroid to treat psoriasis.

Mechanism of Action

Corticosteroids bind to specific receptor proteins and this complex interacts with specific DNA sequences, glucocorticoid response elements, to regulate the expression of corticosteroid-responsive genes. This leads to a myriad of effects, including altered cytokine expression and T cell inhibition.

Topical corticosteroids are available in a wide array of vehicles, including ointments, creams, gels, lotions, powders, shampoos, impregnated tapes (including a recent betamethasone valerate 0.1% occlusive preparation), and more recently sprays and foams. The choice of the vehicle depends on the anatomical sites of the area to be treated. In general, ointments have traditionally been considered to be more effective due to their occlusive nature which leads to enhanced penetration. The addition of propylene glycol increases the solubility of steroids in the vehicle; thus, improving the drug penetration. However, they are greasy in nature and lack cosmetic appeal. Creams are less greasy and less occlusive than ointments, and cosmetically more acceptable to the patients. Hence, creams may be recommended for daytime application, while ointments may be applied at night. Lotions, gels and foams are useful for treating hair-bearing areas, such as the scalp. Foams have been shown to have comparable clinical efficacy to traditional vehicles such as ointments [18]. When applied to the skin, the body heat breaks down the thermolabile foam, depositing the active ingredient directly on the skin. This leads to a higher efficacy and lower systemic toxicity than conventional vehicles. Randomized multicentric double-blinded placebo-controlled trials have also demonstrated efficacy of betamethasone valerate 0.12% foam in scalp psoriasis [19]. One study showed similar results when used for the treatment of non-scalp psoriasis, eliminating the need for separate scalp and body formulations [20]. Clobetasol propionate, when used as a 0.05% measured dose spray, has been shown to be a convenient alternative to traditional preparations. In a recent large-scale community-based 4-week observational study (COBRA trial) of 1,254 patients, clobetasol propionate spray demonstrated excellent efficacy with approximately 90% of patients being satisfied with the treatment [21].

The potency of topical corticosteroids is enhanced by chemical modification of the steroid, e.g. halogenation, methylation and acetylation. Occlusion by applying a hydrocolloid dressing also increases penetration and efficacy [22].

In general, the high-potency corticosteroids are reserved for the treatment of recalcitrant and inflammatory lesions on areas such as elbows, knees, lumbosacral region, palms and soles, with or without occlusion. The lower potency steroids are preferred in thinner skinned areas, such as the face and flexures. To avoid the risk of adverse effects, the weakest corticosteroid that is potentially efficacious should be used, particularly as maintenance therapy.

In clinical practice, especially in the USA, the vast majority of patients are treated initially with high-potency topical corticosteroids. In a study on the use

1 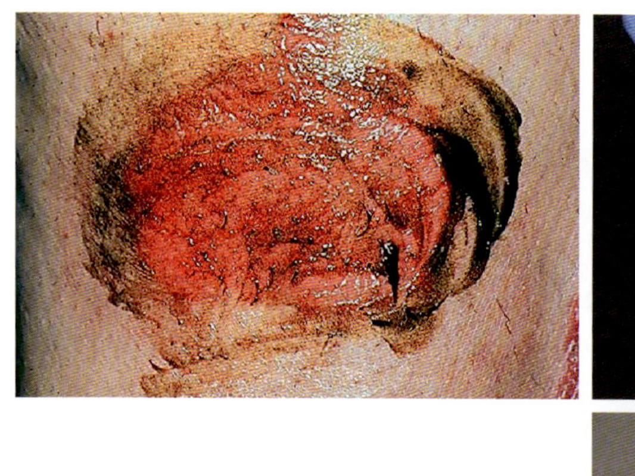

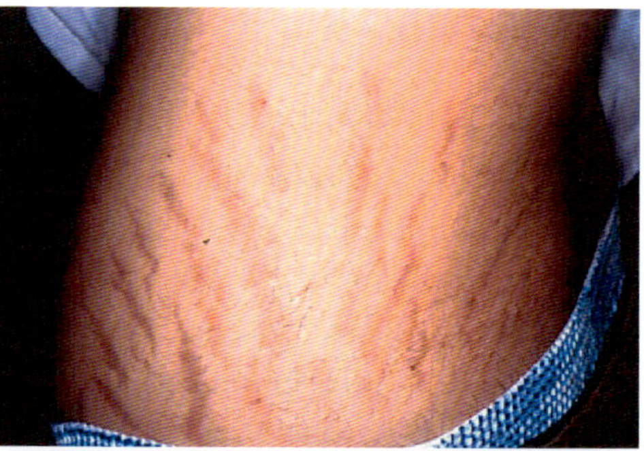 2

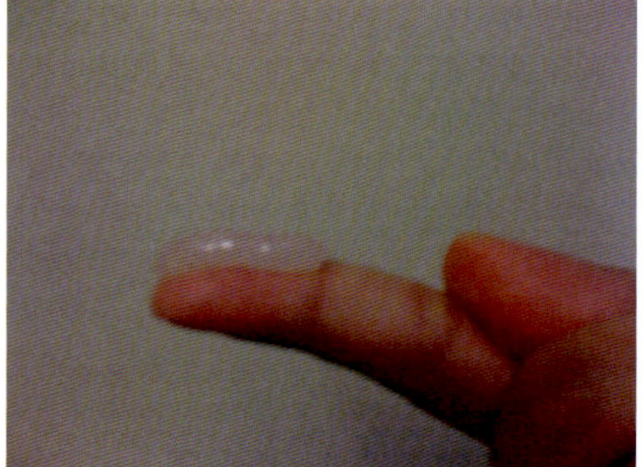 3

Fig. 1. Messiness with tar.
Fig. 2. Striae secondary to topical corticosteroid usage.
Fig. 3. Finger tip unit.

of high-potency corticosteroids in an academic practice [23], it was observed that 79% of patients with psoriasis were prescribed topical corticosteroids, more than half of whom received a high-potency steroid; 11% also received systemic therapy.

Prolonged use of topical corticosteroids is limited by presumed tachyphylaxis, a phenomenon in which medications showing a positive clinical response lose their effectiveness after prolonged use. However, a study designed to identify tachyphylaxis was unable to find any evidence of this phenomenon [24]. In fact, it is now considered that this phenomenon may actually reflect poor adherence to therapy rather than loss of efficacy (see 'Compliance/adherence issues') [25]. To minimize this effect, various innovative regimens have been used. In a weekend therapy in which a super-potent corticosteroid was applied 3 times over a period of 24 h each week, improvement was maintained for up to 6 months in 60% of patients compared with 20% of those who received placebo [26]. Pulse regimens, such as fluticasone twice daily for 2 weeks followed by once daily for 2 days every week for 8 weeks, have been found to be as effective as traditional daily usage while minimizing total steroid exposure [27].

A case report of improvement in rupioid psoriasis, traditionally resistant to topical treatment, with a convenient corticosteroid spray may be an indication that the perceived resistance may be due to poor compliance and not poor penetration [28].

Adverse Effects

Side effects are of concern if topical corticosteroids are used inappropriately or for prolonged periods. Atrophic changes are common and include thinning of the skin, telengiectasias, striae (fig. 2), purpura and easy bruising. Other changes include acneiform changes, perioral dermatitis, rosacea, contact dermatitis, hypertrichosis, pigmentary changes and delayed wound-healing. Fungal infections may be masked, leading to tinea incognito. Certain infections may potentially be aggravated, such as cutaneous candidiasis and herpes simplex.

Systemic side effects are a potential risk if high-potency topical corticosteroids are used over larger surface areas or on thinner areas, such as the face and flexures, for prolonged periods. Children are more susceptible to systemic side effects due to their high surface area to body mass ratio. Side effects include hypothalamus-pituitary axis suppression and iatrogenic Cushing's syndrome.

High-potency corticosteroid application should be therefore limited to a maximum of 50–60 g per week, restricted to <20% of the BSA and used with caution in children. Occlusion with this class of corticosteroids should also be avoided, except on localized individual recalcitrant plaques.

Topical corticosteroids are considered category C drugs during pregnancy. In addition, they are believed to be safe in nursing women provided they are not applied to the nipples and areola.

Recurrence following discontinuation of topical corticosteroid usage is seen in the majority of treated lesions with the mean duration for remission observed to be approximately 2 months [29]. Abrupt withdrawal can also lead to a 'rebound phenomenon' presenting as acute exacerbation of inflammatory psoriasis.

Vitamin D Analogues

Vitamin D_3 was first observed to be beneficial in psoriasis when a patient's psoriasis improved following administration of 1-α hydroxyl vitamin D_3 for treatment of osteoporosis [30]. Calcipotriol (also known as calcipotriene) was the first vitamin D analogue to be used in psoriasis. Subsequently, calcitriol (1,25 dihyroxy vitamin D_3) and tacalcitol were developed, with maxacalcitol and tisocalcitate most recently added to the armamentarium. Only calcipotriol is currently available in the USA (table 1). Vitamin D analogues have now become a first-line treatment for plaque psoriasis, being more cosmetically acceptable and efficacious than older treatments like tar and dithranol, and of equal potency to the mid-high range of potency of topical corticosteroids.

steroid-sparing agent while the steroid minimizes the irritancy potential of calcipotriol, leading to an improvement in quality of life measures. The combination therapy is safe and well tolerated, as observed by a large-scale 52-week randomized safety study, when used on its own or alternating with calcipotriol alone [37]. The addition of calcipotriol twice daily on weekdays to a weekend pulse therapy of superpotent corticosteroids has been observed to increase the duration of remission [38]. Likewise, a combination of corticosteroid in the morning and vitamin D analogue at night followed by maintenance with the vitamin D analogue alone has also been shown to be effective in clinical trials [39].

Calcipotriol has also been tried in combination with phototherapy and photochemotherapy with mixed results. A multicenter randomized controlled trial showed that twice-weekly UVB in combination with calcipotriol was equal in efficacy to thrice-weekly UVB alone while requiring fewer UVB exposures [40]. However, a meta-analysis revealed no significant beneficial effect of the combination when compared with UVB alone [41]. On the other hand, addition of calcipotriol to PUVA has clearly demonstrated increased efficacy and reduction in the number of UVA exposures and cumulative dose. Calcipotriol must be applied after UVA exposure since irradiation with UVA inactivates it [42].

A meta-analysis of studies using calcipotriene with oral acitretin demonstrated increased efficacy of the combination over acitretin monotherapy; clearance can be achieved with a lower cumulative dose of acitretin [41]. The addition of calcipotriol to cyclosporine A has also shown the combination to be more effective than monotherapy [43].

Topical Retinoids

Retinoids are vitamin A derivatives which modulate epidermal proliferation, and have been used systemically for psoriasis for nearly 3 decades. Tazarotene is a synthetic acetylenic retinoid and was the first topical retinoid approved for the management of psoriasis, being available as 0.05% and 0.1% gel and cream formulations.

Mechanism of Action

Tazarotene is a prodrug and is rapidly metabolized to its active metabolite tazarotenic acid. It acts by binding to retinoid receptors RAR-β/γ with little affinity for the RXR receptors. The combination binds to specific sites which regulate the transcription of genes involved in the pathogenesis of psoriasis. Three tazarotene-induced genes have been identified which are involved in epidermal proliferation and differentiation, namely TIG 1, 2 and 3. Tazarotene modulates the pathogenesis of psoriasis through 3 mechanisms, namely: reduction in keratinocyte proliferation, normalization of keratinocyte differentiation and a decrease in expression of inflammatory mediators.

A large placebo-controlled study indicated that 0.05 or 1% gel gave a 50% reduction in PASI score after 12 weeks [44]. Double-blind randomized controlled trials have indicated similar efficacy. An added advantage with the use of tazarotene is its ability to maintain clinical benefits for up to 12 weeks after discontinuation of therapy [45].

Tazarotene is comparable in efficacy to mid-potency steroids, but weaker than super-potent steroids [46].

Adverse Effects

Topical tazarotene's major side effect is dose-dependent local irritation, erythema and burning, and is therefore not recommended for application on sensitive areas, such as the face and flexures. Irritation can be minimized by the use of cream formulations, lower concentrations, application on alternate days and combination with topical corticosteroids. Short-contact application for 20 min appears to be as effective, while irritation is less frequent or less severe.

The systemic bioavailability following topical application is low (about 1%), and thus minimizing potential systemic side effects. However, tazarotene is categorized as a category X drug, and should not be prescribed in pregnant or lactating females. A baseline pregnancy test before prescribing tazarotene has been advocated.

Combination Therapy

The combination of topical corticosteroids with tazarotene has enhanced efficacy and lessened irritation as compared with tazarotene monotherapy. The clearance is more rapid and the period of remission is longer [47]. In addition, tazarotene may also prevent corticosteroid-induced atrophy [48].

Tazarotene can be combined with either broadband or narrowband UVB as it is photostable. However, it can result in thinning of the stratum corneum, allowing the patients to burn more easily. A 2-week course of tazarotene decreases the minimal erythema dose of UVB by about 25%; therefore, doses of UVB should be reduced accordingly. The addition of tazarotene to narrowband UVB leads to a more rapid and effective clearing of psoriasis compared to narrowband UVB alone [49].

Tazarotene and PUVA baths have been found to be clinically superior to PUVA alone. The UVA dose required to induce immediate pigment darkening is also reduced by about 8% when used in combination with tazarotene; therefore, PUVA should be initiated at lower doses [50]. No significant phototoxicity has been noted with tazarotene.

Bexarotene (Tagretin®) is an RXR-selective retinoid which binds to RXR receptors, and therefore is sometimes referred to as 'rexinoid'. It is currently approved for the treatment of cutaneous T cell lymphoma and has been studied in psoriasis, both orally and topically as a 1% gel, with limited data available regarding its efficacy. Bexarotene has been combined with narrowband UVB, and was shown to be more effective than narrowband UVB with placebo. However, large-scale studies are needed to clearly demonstrate the beneficial role of this agent.

Calcineurin Inhibitors

Calcineurin inhibitors are macrolide immunosuppressants, and include tacrolimus, pimecrolimus, and sirolimus.

Mechanism of Action

Tacrolimus (FK506) binds to a specific binding protein (FKBP); this complex then binds and inhibits calcineurin. Calcineurin is therefore unable to dephosphorylate NFAT (nuclear factor of activate T cells) which is a transcription factor involved in the regulation of expression of genes coding for inflammatory cytokines.

When used systemically, they have been documented to show substantial efficacy in psoriasis. As a topical application, tacrolimus is available as 0.03 and 1% ointment and pimecrolimus is available as 1% ointment with limited data supporting their efficacy with topical use. The first trials of topical tacrolimus failed to demonstrate efficacy in chronic plaque psoriasis [51]. However, it was shown to be effective when used under occlusion or on the thinner skin of the face or flexures [52]. Used under occlusion, it has been found to be superior to calcitriol, but less efficacious than calcipotriol. While occlusion increases efficacy, it may also increase the frequency and intensity of side effects.

Efficacy, even in the most severe cases, suggests that topical calcineurin inhibitors may be the treatment of choice for these 2 areas.

A double-blind randomized vehicle-controlled study in patients with moderate to severe intertriginous psoriasis comparing twice daily application of 1% pimecrolimus versus its vehicle showed a rapid and significant response to the drug along with an excellent tolerability [53]. Its use did not induce skin atrophy or secondary skin infections.

Adverse Effects

These include burning, erythema and stinging. Systemic side effects have not been reported even with large BSA applications. However, large-scale studies are needed to establish safety following topical application. Similarly, although studies have suggested efficacy as well as safety in children and elderly, long-term studies are necessary. Topical calcineurin inhibitors are not currently approved for the treatment of psoriasis.

Concerns have been raised about the development of skin cancers and lymphoma with these agents, as suggested by animal studies and rare case reports. While the association remains to be clearly established, the FDA has issued a public health advisory regarding its use, particularly for long-term administration and in children less than 2 years old.

Sirolimus (rapamycin) is described in the section 'Future of topical therapy'.

Compliance/Adherence Issues

Adherence to therapy remains a major challenge in the management of psoriasis, especially in the area of topical therapy. The term 'adherence' has now replaced the prior term 'compliance' as compliance suggests a negative impression in which a patient passively follows physician's orders. Poor adherence can be anticipated in the management of chronic disorders such as psoriasis, with studies revealing that less than half the patients actually follow the physician's recommendations [54]. While one may assume adherence to be directly proportional to the severity of psoriasis, studies have revealed that intentional non-adherence was more likely in patients with severe psoriasis as determined by the physical extent of the disease or impact on the quality of life [55].

Factors that influence adherence include disease-related issues (e.g. extent of the disease), patient characteristics (e.g. age, with elderly patients being generally more compliant than younger ones), gender, personal beliefs, socio-cultural factors, and treatment characteristics (e.g. complexity of usage of treatment, cost, efficacy). However, no consistent factors have been found which can predict adherence. Even though adherence to treatment is of vital importance to its effectiveness, relatively few studies have been carried out to study effective strategies to improve adherence. The physician-patient relationship is thus critical for better adherence to therapy. Proper patient education, clear instructions about usage of the drug, information about potential side effects, simple and less-frequent dosing, and convenient treatment protocols which minimally interfere with patient's lifestyle may all help achieve better adherence. Adherence also tends to increase around the time of physician visits, a phenomenon termed as the 'white coat effect', suggesting that regularly scheduled visits are likely to help improve adherence to therapy.

The usage of the concept of finger tip unit (FTU) may help patients better dose their topical treatment. An FTU is the amount of cream/ointment expressed from a 5-mm nozzle applied from the distal skin crease to the tip of the patient's index finger (fig. 3). One FTU is estimated to be approximately 500 mg while approximately 30–40 g are required for whole body application. Thus, the number of FTU required for each affected body site can be calculated accordingly (table 2). Inclusion of clear FTU instructions along with images and a chart to show the number of units required for specific areas of the body could help improve the patient's understanding of the therapy, thereby improving adherence and response to therapy [56].

Table 2. BSA percentage

Area to be treated	Approximate BSA, %	FTU required (approx.), n
Scalp	6	3
Face	3	1.5
Palms	2	1
Hands (front and back)	4	2
Both arms (including hands)	9	4.5
Elbows (large plaque)	2	1
Soles	3	1.5
Feet (dorsum and sole)	6	3
Both legs including feet	32	16
Buttocks	8	4
Knees (large plaque)	2	1
Trunk (anterior)	16	8
Trunk (posterior)	16	8
Genitalia	1	0.5

Future of Topical Therapy

New Topical Vitamin D Analogues

Calcipotriol, calcitriol and tacalcitol are currently available in Europe, while in the USA the only vitamin D analogue approved for use in psoriasis is calcipotriol. Considering the potential benefits and improved adverse effect profile in comparison to corticosteroid therapy, extensive research has been carried out in the development of new vitamin D analogues which have a similar or higher efficacy than the traditional ones while having a better side effect profile. These may represent the next-generation vitamin D analogues to be used in the topical treatment of psoriasis.

Maxacalcitol was found to have about 10 times greater efficacy than calcipotriol in suppressing keratinocyte proliferation in vitro. A double-blind placebo-controlled randomized left-versus-right concentration-response study was performed with once-daily application of maxacalcitol in patients with mild to moderate chronic plaque psoriasis [57]. All concentrations of maxacalcitol ointment (6, 12.5, 25 and 50 μg/g) were observed to have clinical efficacy as compared to placebo, with the greatest efficacy being noted at 25 μg/g by week 2. Improvement continued throughout the study period without a plateau effect by week 8, suggesting a beneficial effect of a longer duration of therapy. When compared to calcipotriol, maxacalcitol appeared to more effective. Although no systemic side effects were noted, long-term usage or large BSA application would be needed to assess its effect on calcium metabolism.

Double-blind placebo-controlled randomized inter-individual studies on a newly developed vitamin D analogue, tisocalcitate, have demonstrated safety from systemic side effects and better skin tolerability when applied as a 50 μg/g ointment over 45% BSA in healthy volunteers [58].

Paricalcitol, a vitamin D analogue used in patients with renal insufficiency, has been studied for its potential in the management of psoriasis. A double-blind randomized right-left-comparison placebo-controlled study demonstrated a moderate to excellent response in patients receiving the drug [59]. The therapy was found to be well tolerated with no significant changes in calcium or phosphorous levels.

Becocalcidiol is another recently described topical vitamin D analogue. A multicenter double-blind vehicle-controlled randomized controlled trial was carried out comparing becocalcidiol (75 μg/g once or twice daily) versus placebo for 8 weeks [60]. Becocalcidiol demonstrated efficacy with about 25% of patients showing almost complete clearing of the lesions. The drug was very well tolerated, with only a quarter experiencing mild skin irritation and pruritus. Hypercalcemia or hypercalciuria was not observed in any of the patients.

New Calcineurin Inhibitors

Sirolimus (rapamycin) is a newer topical calcineurin inhibitor recently tested for use in psoriasis [61]. Following its documented efficacy when used systemically, a double-blind left-versus-right randomized study was carried out, with doses of 2.2 and 8% sirolimus ointment. Immunohistochemical assessment of the lesions showed significant improvement with topical sirolimus, as did the clinical scores. Poor penetration could be an issue, which may be resolved by using it under occlusion. Large-scale studies are warranted to confirm its efficacy and safety.

New Formulations

Novel Liposomal Dithranol

Enhanced penetration and efficacy were noted when dithranol was used in a vehicle containing liposomes. Recently, a formulation has been developed which contains dithranol 'entrapped in phospholipid liposomes'. A randomized double-blind vehicle-controlled within-patient comparison study was carried out using 0.5% dithranol lipogel on one side and pure liposomal base or conventional dithranol cream on the other side [62]. The liposome-entrapped formulation demonstrated comparable efficacy to the conventional cream formulation along with markedly low irritation and minimal staining, suggesting these new formulations may hold promise for an upsurge in the use of dithranol in future.

There has been extensive research into the use of systemic drugs as topical preparations to limit the occurrence of systemic adverse effects. Topical applications must be designed while evaluating the characteristics of the active ingredient, such as molecular size, lipid solubility, stability in the vehicle, concentration in various cells in the skin and systemic absorption.

Methotrexate, a folate antagonist, has been used systemically in the management of psoriasis since 1971 with well-documented clinical efficacy. In an attempt to avoid side effects, such as gastrointestinal irritation, hepatotoxicity and bone marrow suppression, methotrexate has been tried topically for decades. Early studies failed to show any efficacy [63], attributable mainly to lack of penetration of the stratum corneum by the drug when used in a cream form. As methotrexate is a water-soluble drug with high molecular weight and dissolution at physiological pH, different modes of delivery have been attempted, including penetration enhancers such as decylmethyl sulfoxide, laurocapram, propylene glycol and isopropyl alcohol. Use of methotrexate at a concentration of 0.25% and 1% in a hydrophilic gel has been found to be clinically effective and well tolerated [64, 65]. In vitro studies have revealed that delivery from microemulsion was even better than delivery from aqueous solutions of the drug [66]. Optimal therapeutic skin concentrations of methotrexate remain to be delineated, and further studies will hopefully allow for ascertainment of the maximally effective topical dose.

Drugs can be delivered into the skin by a technique known as iontophoresis, involving the use of a direct current to increase the penetration of ionic drugs to a limited area. It has been tried in the delivery of large ionic molecules such as local anesthetics, antiperspirants and antineoplastic agents.

Electroporation is another method of improving drug delivery involving application of an ultrashort electric pulse to break down the permeability barrier, during which large molecules can pass through local transport regions. Animal studies using electroporation along with concurrent iontophoresis, lipid enhancers and local hyperthermia led to delivery of a significant amount of methotrexate through intact skin within a short application time.

Intralesional Therapy

Intralesional treatments, delivering a high dose of medication to a localized area, have long been used in psoriasis with insoluble preparations such as triamcinolone acetonide (10 mg/ml) and triamcinolone hexacetonide (10 mg/ml). These agents solubilize gradually, and therefore have a prolonged duration of action with minimal systemic toxicity and a prolonged duration of action. This therapy has specifically been used for the management of nail psoriasis, injecting the drug into the nail matrix where topical agents fail to gain access easily. The procedure is inevitably painful with pericuticular atrophy being a problem.

Other intralesional drugs which have been tried in the past include cyclosporine and 5-flouro-uracil for localized plaques of psoriasis.

Conclusion

Topical therapy is likely to remain the mainstay of therapy for the majority of patients with psoriasis. Despite over a century of use and a wide variety of available agents and formulations internationally, specific recommendations and high-quality clinical studies are proportionally surprisingly few. The vexed questions of adherence to therapy, tachyphylaxis, combination therapies and the use of specific agents for specific anatomical sites remain to be more formally evaluated. Finally, patient education is paramount, and time spent by all clinicians in this endeavor will certainly be rewarded by better clinical outcomes.

References

1 Menter A, Griffiths CEM: Current and future management of psoriasis. Lancet 2007;370:272–284.

2 Fredrickson T, Petterson U: Severe psoriasis: oral therapy with a new retinoid. Dermatologica 1978; 157:238–244.

3 Langley RG, Ellis CN: Evaluating psoriasis with Psoriasis Area and Severity Index, Psoriasis Global Assessment, and Lattice System Physician's Global Assessment. J Am Acad Dermatol 2004;51:563–569.

4 Finlay AY: Current severe psoriasis and the rule of tens. Br J Dermatol 2005;152:861–867.

5 Berth-Jones J, Thompson J, Papp K: A study examining inter-rater and intra-rater reliability of a novel instrument for assessment of psoriasis: the Copenhagen Psoriasis Severity Index. Br J Dermatol 2008;159:407–412.

6 Koo J, Cuffie CA, Tanner DJ, Bressinck R, Cornell RC, DeVillez RL, Edwards L, Breneman DL, Piacquadio DJ, Guzzo CA, Monroe EW: Mometasone furoate 0.1%-salicylic acid 5% ointment in the treatment of moderate-to-severe psoriasis: a multicenter study. Clin Ther 1998;20:283–291.

7 Kuokkanen K, Zador G: A double blind comparison of betamethasone dipropionate with salicylic acid (Diprosalic®) and budesonide ointment in the treatment of psoriasis. Curr Ther Res 1983;34:459–468.

8 Carroll CL, Clarke J, Camacho F, Balkrishnan R, Feldman SR: Topical tacrolimus ointment combined with 6% salicylic acid gel for plaque psoriasis treatment. Arch Dermatol 2005;141:43–46.

9 Goeckerman WH: Treatment of psoriasis. Northwest Med 1925;24:229–231.

10 Goodfield M, Kownacki S, Berth-Jones J: Double-blind randomized, multicentre, parallel group study comparing a 1% coal tar preparation (Exorex) with a 5% coal tar preparation (Alphosyl) in chronic plaque psoriasis. J Dermatol Treat 2004;15:14–22.

11 Gawkrodger DJ, Therapy Guidelines and Audit Subcommittee of the British Association of Dermatologists: Current management of psoriasis. J Dermatol Treat 1997;8:27–55.

12 McGill A, Frank A, Emmett N, Turnbull DM, Birch-Machin MA, Reynolds NJ: The anti-psoriatic drug anthralin accumulates in keratinocyte mitochondria, dissipates mitochondrial membrane potential, and induces apoptosis through a pathway dependent on respiratory competent mitochondria. FASEB J 2005;19:1012–1014.

13 Ingram JT: The approach to psoriasis. BMJ 1953;2: 591–594.
14 Schaefer H, Farber EM, Goldberg L, Schalla W: Limited application period for dithranol in psoriasis: preliminary report on penetration and clinical efficacy. Br J Dermatol 1989;102:571–573.
15 Ramsay B, Lawrence CM, Bruce JM, Shuster S: The effects of triethanolamine application on anthralin-induced inflammation and therapeutic effect in psoriasis. J Am Acad Dermatol 1990;23:73–76.
16 Gerritsen MJ, Boezeman JB, Elbers ME, van de Kerkhof PCM: Dithranol embedded in crystalline monoglycerides combined with phototherapy (UVB): a new approach in the treatment of psoriasis. Skin Pharmacol Appl Skin Physiol 1998;11:133–139.
17 Cornell RC, Stoughton RB: Correlation of the vasoconstriction assay and clinical activity in psoriasis. Arch Dermatol 1985;121:63–67.
18 Feldman SR, Sangha N, Setaluri V: Topical corticosteroid in foam vehicle offers comparable coverage compared with traditional vehicles. J Am Acad Dermatol 2000;42:1017–1020.
19 Franz TJ, Parsell DA, Halualani RM, Hannigan JF, Kalbach JP, Harkonen WS: Betamethasone valerate foam 0.12%: a novel vehicle with enhanced delivery and efficacy. Int J Dermatol 1999;38:628–632.
20 Lebwohl M, Sherer D, Washenik K, Krueger GG, Menter A, Koo J, Feldman SR: A randomized, double-blind, placebo-controlled study of clobetasol propionate 0.05% foam in the treatment of nonscalp psoriasis. Int J Dermatol 2002;41:269–274.
21 Menter A: Topical monotherapy with clobetasol propionate spray 0.05% in the COBRA trial. Cutis 2007;80:12–19.
22 Volden G, Kragbelle K, van de Kerkhof PC, Aberg K, White RJ: Remission and relapse of chronic plaque psoriasis treated once a week with clobetasol propionate occluded with a hydrocolloid dressing versus twice daily treatment with clobetasol propionate alone. J Dermatol Treat 2001;12:141–144.
23 Pearce DJ, Spencer L, Hu J, Balkrishnan R, Fleisher AB Jr, Feldman SR: Class I topical corticosteroid use by psoriasis patients in an academic practice. J Dermatolog Treat 2004;15:235–238.
24 Miller JJ, Roling D, Margolis D, Guzzo C: Failure to demonstrate therapeutic tachyphylaxis to topically applied steroids in patients with psoriasis. J Am Acad Dermatol 1999;41:546–549.
25 Feldman SR: Tachyphylaxis to topical corticosteroids: the more you use them, the less they work? Clin Dermatol 2006;24:229–230.
26 Katz HI, Prawer SE,Medansky RS, Krueger GG, Mooney JJ, Jones ML, et al: Intermittent corticosteroid maintenance treatment of psoriasis: a double-blind multicenter trial of augmented betamethasone dipropionate ointment in a pulse dose treatment regimen. Dermatologica 1991;183:269–274.
27 Lebwohl M, Tan MH, Meador SL, Singer G: Limited application of fluticasone propionate ointment, 0.005% in patients with psoriasis of the face and intertriginous areas. J Am Acad Dermatol 2001;44: 77–82.
28 Feldman SR, Brown KL, Heald P: 'Coral reef' psoriasis: a marker of resistance to topical treatment. J Dermatol Treat 2008;30:1–2.
29 Koo J, Lebwohl M: Duration of remission of psoriasis therapies. J Am Acad Dermatol 1999;41:51–59.
30 Morimoto S, Kumahara Y: A patient with psoriasis cured by 1 alpha-hydroxyvitamin D_3. Med J Osaka Univ 1985;35:51–54.
31 Lu I, Gilleadeau P, McLane JA, Heftler N, Kamber M, Gottlieb S, Krueger JG, Gottlieb AB: Modulation of epidermal differentiation, tissue inflammation, and T-lymphocyte infiltration in psoriatic plaques by topical calcitriol. J Cutan Pathol 1996;23:419–430.
32 Dubertret L, Wallach D, Souteyrand P, Perussel M, Kalis B, Meynadier J, Chevrant-Breton J, Beylot C, Bazex JA, Jurgensen HJ: Efficacy and safety of calcipotriol (MC 903) ointment in psoriasis vulgaris: a randomized, double-blind, right/left comparative, vehicle-controlled study. J Am Acad Dermatol 1992; 27:983–988.
33 Gerritsen MJ, van de Kerkhof PCM, Langner A: Long-term safety of topical calcitriol 3 microg g(−1) ointment. Br J Dermatol 2001;144(suppl 58): 17–19.
34 van de Kerkhof PC, Werfel T, Haustein UF, et al: Tacalcitol ointment in the treatment of psoriasis vulgaris: a multicentre, placebo-controlled, double-blind study on efficacy and safety. Br J Dermatol 2002;135:758–765.
35 Scarpa C: Tacalcitol ointment is an efficacious and well tolerated treatment for psoriasis. J Eur Acad Dermatol Venereol 1996;6:142–146.
36 Camarasa JM, Ortonne JP, Dubertret L: Calcitriol shows greater persistence of treatment effect than betamethasone diproprionate in topical psoriasis therapy. J Dermatol Treat 2003;14:8–13.
37 Kragballe K, Austad J, Barnes L et al: A 52-week randomized safety study of calcipotriol/betamethasone dipropionate two-compound product in the treatment of psoriasis. Br J Dermatol 2006;154:1150–1160.

38 Lebwohl M, Yoles A, Lombardi K, Lou W: Calcipotriene ointment and halobetasol ointment in the long-term treatment of psoriasis: effects on the duration of improvement. J Am Acad Dermatol 1998;39:447–450.
39 Lahfa M, Mrowietz U, Koenig M, Simon JC: Calcitriol ointment and clobetasol propionate cream: a new regimen for the treatment of plaque psoriasis. Eur J Dermatol 2003;13:261–265.
40 Ramsay CA, Schwartz BE, Lowson D, Papp K, Bolduc A, Gilbert M: Calcipotriol cream combined with twice weekly broad-band UVB phototherapy: a safe, effective and UVB-sparing antipsoriatric combination treatment. The Canadian Calcipotriol and UVB Study Group. Dermatology 2000;200:17–24.
41 Ashcroft DM, Li Wan Po A, Williams HC, Griffiths CE: Combination regimens of topical calcipotriene in chronic plaque psoriasis: systematic review of efficacy and tolerability. Arch Dermatol 2000;136: 1536–1543.
42 Lebwohl M, Hecker D, Martinez J, Sapadin A, Patel B: Interactions between calcipotriene and ultraviolet light. J Am Acad Dermatol 1997;37:93–95.
43 Grossman RM, Thivolet J, Claudy A, Souteyrand P, Guilhou J, Thomas P, et al: A novel therapeutic approach to psoriasis with combination calcipotriol ointment and very low-dose cyclosporine: results of a multicenter placebo-controlled study. J Am Acad Dermatol 1994;31:68–74.
44 Weinstein GD, Krueger GG, Lowe NJ, et al: Tazarotene gel, a new retinoid, for topical therapy of psoriasis: vehicle-controlled study of safety, efficacy, and duration of therapeutic effect. J Am Acad Dermatol 1997;37:85–92.
45 Weinstein GD: Tazarotene gel: efficacy and safety in plaque psoriasis. J Am Acad Dermatol 1997; 37(suppl):S33–S38.
46 Lebwohl M: Psoriasis. Lancet 2003;361:1197–1204.
47 Koo JYM, Martin D: Investigator-masked comparison of tazarotene gel q.d. plus mometasone furoate cream q.d. vs. mometasone furoate cream b.i.d. in the treatment of plaque psoriasis. Int J Dermatol 2001;40:210–212.
48 Lebwohl MG, Breneman DL, Goffe BS, Grossman JR, Ling MR, Milbauer J, Pincus SH, Sibbald RG, Swinyer LJ, Weinstein D, Lew-Kaya DA, Lue JC, Gibson JR, Sefton J: Tazarotene 0.1% gel plus corticosteroid cream in the treatment of plaque psoriasis. J Am Acad Dermatol 1998;39:590–596.
49 Behrens S, Grundmann-Kollmann M, Scheiner R, Peter RU, Kerscher M: Combination phototherapy of psoriasis with narrow-band UVB irradiation and topical tazarotene gel. J Am Acad Dermatol 200;42: 493–495.
50 Hecker D, Worsely J, Yueh G, Kuroda K, Lebwohl M: Interactions between tazarotene and ultraviolet light. J Am Acad Dermatol 1999;41:927–930.
51 Zonneveld IM, Rubins A, Jablonska S, Dobozy A, Ruzika T, Kind P, Dubertret L, Bos JD, et al: Topical tacrolimus is not effective in chronic plaque psoriasis: a pilot study. Arch Dermatol 1998;134:1101–1102.
52 Lebwohl M, Freeman AK, Chapman MS, Feldman SR, Hartle JE, Henning A, Tacrolimus Ointment study group: Tacrolimus ointment is effective for facial and intertriginous psoriasis. J Am Acad Dermatol 2004;51:723–730.
53 Gribetz C, Ling M, Lebwohl M, et al: Pimecrolimus cream 1% in the treatment of intertriginous psoriasis: a double-blind, randomised study. J Am Acad Dermatol 2004;51:731–738.
54 Richards HL, Fortune DG, O'Sullivan TM, Main CJ, Griffiths CE: Patients with psoriasis and their compliance with medication. J Am Acad Dermatol 1999; 41:581–583.
55 Zaghloul SS, Goodfield MJ: Objective assessment of compliance with psoriasis treatment. Arch Dermatol 2004;140:408–414.
56 Bewley A, Dermatology working group: Expert consensus: time for a change in the way we advise our patients to use topical corticosteroids. Br J Dermatol 2008;158:917–920.
57 Barker JN, Ashton RE, Marks R, Harris RI, Berth Jones J: Topical maxacalcitol for the treatment of psoriasis vulgaris: a placebo-controlled, double-blind, dose-finding study with active comparator. Br J Dermatol 1999;141:274–278.
58 Schneider M, Staks T, Jahreis A, O'Keefe E: Safety of large area application of a novel vitamin D analogue (Tisocalcitate ointment) in patients with chronic plaque type psoriasis. J Am Acad Dermatol 2004; 50(suppl 1):179.
59 Durakovic C, Ray S, Holick MF: Topical paricalcitol (19-nor-1 alpha,25-dihydroxyvitamin D_2) is a novel, safe and effective treatment for plaque psoriasis: a pilot study. Br J Dermatol 2004;151:190–195.
60 Helfrich YR, Kang S, Hamilton TA, Voorhees JJ: Topical becocalcidiol for the treatment of psoriasis vulgaris: a randomized, placebo-controlled, double-blind, multicentre study. Br J Dermatol 2007;157: 369–374.

topical therapy is insufficient. Patients with >3–5% body surface area (BSA) affected are considered to have moderate psoriasis, and patients with >10% BSA affected are considered to have severe disease. Phototherapy may be a first-line treatment option in these patients due to its efficacy and systemic safety profile. Phototherapy is also an excellent option for patients with other medical problems, for whom systemic medications including cyclosporine, methotrexate, and the biological agents may not be suitable.

NB-UVB Phototherapy

NB-UVB may be a useful treatment modality not only for treatment-resistant patients and patients for whom other therapies are contraindicated, but also as a first- or second-line agent in the treatment of psoriasis. NB-UVB has been utilized extensively throughout Europe, Asia, Australia, and the USA. Ultraviolet B light lies between visible light and X-rays on the electromagnetic spectrum, ranging from 290 to 320 nm. NB-UVB uses only a limited range of this spectrum, emitting a distinct narrow band of high-intensity light from 311 to 313 nm. This helps eliminate high-energy shorter wavelengths responsible for burning, premature aging, and increased incidence of skin cancer. Based on early studies from the 1980s, the 313-nm wavelength allows for the lowest effective dosage of light with the least erythema and the optimal therapeutic effect [1, 2].

Efficacy

To induce steady improvement of existing psoriatic lesions, outpatient UVB phototherapy should be performed at least 3 times weekly. If UVB phototherapy is conducted less than 3 times per week, the rate of clinical improvement diminishes significantly. In an average patient with scattered plaque-type psoriasis, at least 20–30 UVB treatment sessions are required to induce significant improvement or clearance. The Leone Dermatology Center in Chicago, which established a NB-UVB dosing protocol based on skin typing, estimates the number of treatments to clear a patient is between 30 and 35 sessions. In the clinical experience of the authors, the success rate for basic UVB phototherapy ranges from 50 to 80%. With NB-UVB, most patients show significant improvement or clearance of trunk lesions. If one makes an allowance for residual lesions on the elbows, knees, and shins, approximately 80% of the patients can be considered to be successfully treated. Patients should be treated for approximaely 3 months, followed by maintenance therapy. The authors recommend that maintenance therapy consists of NB-UVB treatments 1–2 times weekly, which can range from months to years depending on the specific patient and disease course. Significant reduction in scaling may be noted after the first 3–6 treatments, and a significant response seen after 6–9 treatments.

For the treatment of psoriasis, multiple studies have shown NB-UVB to be more effective than BB-UVB [3–6]. However, NB-UVB requires higher dosages of light to achieve minimal erythema, and thus requires longer treatment times when compared to BB-UVB [3–8]. To compensate for higher required light dosages, NB-UVB boxes are sold containing 24–48 bulbs to help shorten treatment times. Several reports indicate that less aggressive NB-UVB regimens with shorter treatment times are just as efficacious in clearing psoriasis [1, 9–11].

In a recent study evaluating both PUVA and NB-UVB in patients with skin types I-IV, 65% of patients achieved clearance using NB-UVB and 35% of patients who cleared with NB-UVB maintained clearance for 6 months, without any further phototherapy treatments [12]. Patients were treated with NB-UVB twice weekly until clearance or until a maximum of 30 sessions. The median number of treatments to clearance was 28.5 treatments in the NB-UVB group. Examining the data, NB-UVB is generally more effective than PUVA in clearing trunk psoriasis while PUVA is generally more effective than NB-UVB in clearing plaques on the extremities. Regarding remission, in one study, the authors reported a remission rate of 38% approximately 1 year after cessation of therapy [7]. The average time to relapse was 3 months for the remaining 62% of patients.

Safety

Similar to other phototherapies, side effects of NB-UVB include erythema and blistering. In one study, compared to PUVA, a greater proportion of patients developed erythema, but PUVA-treated patients were more likely to miss treatments due to burning, reflecting the long-lasting nature of PUVA erythema [13]. Some studies find more damaging potential of NB-UVB when 2.0 minimal erythema dose (MED) is exceeded, based on the number of necrotic keratinocytes in histopathological sections of skin [3]. With NB-UVB therapy, there have also been reports of rare blistering strictly at the site of psoriatic lesions while the surrounding skin remains unaffected [14–16]. Some have speculated that due to rapid clearance by NB-UVB, psoriatic plaques may not gain the same photoprotection as normal skin, exposing them to a burning dose midway through treatment [16].

In patients treated with long-term BB-UVB, there is essentially no increased risk of skin cancer [17]. Murine experiments examining carcinogenicity offer conflicting data depending on mouse strains used, light dosage, and treatment schedules. Most long-term epidemiological studies examining patients on UVB phototherapy for 2 decades failed to show any increase in skin cancer rates compared to the general population [18–20]. Studies which did demonstrate increased carcinogenesis also had higher rates of burning [21]. In clinical practice, adjusting the dosage of light to limit burning may be the key to limiting carcinogenesis of NB-UVB, since lower-dosage regimens are as effective as high-dosage regimens [10]. Regarding patients with a personal history of non-melanoma skin cancer, phototherapy is considered a suitable treatment option; however, other non-phototherapy treatment options should be sought if the patient has a history of multiple non-melanoma skin cancers. For patients with a history of melanoma, other treatment options including systemic agents and topical treatments should be considered, although a history of melanoma does not strictly preclude the use of phototherapy.

UVB phototherapy is contraindicated in patients taking photosensitizing medications, including thiazide diuretics, loop diuretics, specific antibiotics, antidepressants, and antipsychotics. However, it is possible to conduct phototherapy after exposing a test area of skin to UVB light without a reaction. This negative result of MED testing can help prove that the particular patient is not experiencing photosensitivity from the 'photosensitizing' medication. UVB phototherapy is contraindicated in patients with photosensitizing diseases, such as lupus erythematosus or polymorphous light eruption, unless phototherapy is utilized specifically to harden the skin.

NB-UVB is considered safe and well-tolerated in pregnant women and children; however, long-term data regarding carcinogenic potential and adverse effects in children undergoing NB-UVB phototherapy is lacking. Additionally, practitioners have not noticed widespread adverse reactions to NB-UVB phototherapy in HIV-infected patients. In published research, there have been no described changes in immune function among HIV-positive patients undergoing UVB phototherapy [22]. Most practitioners consider UVB phototherapy safer than modalities such as PUVA, methotrexate, and cyclosporine.

Dosage and Administration

There are 2 regimens currently available for treating patients with NB-UVB. The first involves determining a patient's MED [23]. This requires patch testing with varying quantities of light to determine the dosage that produces just perceptible erythema 24 h after irradiation. UVB phototherapy tends to produce maximal results when used at or near a patient's MED, but this erythemogenic schedule is not practical because many patients experience uncomfortable burning sensations at MED, and practitioners do not want to risk burning patients [24, 25]. The alternative is a suberythemogenic schedule where the initial dosage of UVB light is some percentage of the MED, which minimizes the cumulative dosage of UVB radiation and the risk of inducing UVB burns. Typically, first exposures start at 70% of the MED. Subsequent exposures given 3 times weekly are determined based on the reaction to the previous treatment. MED determination is tedious and time-consuming, and therefore most clinicians do not do it. For those who do, Phillips make a 7-inch twin tube lamp for which Daavlin has designed a handheld unit, which can be used as a MED tester.

In a high-volume practice, formal MED testing can be quite labor intensive and disruptive to the flow of patients undergoing phototherapy. Instead, our clinic uses

Table 1. Narrow-band skin type-based dosing protocol, established by the Leone Dermatology Center

Skin type	Initial dose, mJ	Subsequent increase in dose, mJ	Estimated goal range, mJ
I	130	15	520
II	220	25	880
III	260	40	1,040
IV	330	45	1,320
V	350	60	1,400
VI	400	65	1,600
Vitiligo	170	30	680

Reprinted from Shelk and Morgan [26], with permission from the publisher.

a defined guideline to determine the starting dosage for NB-UVB therapy based on skin typing (table 1). The Leone Dermatology Center in Chicago has established this percentage-based protocol based on skin type, using National Biological Corporation equipment [26]. Patients are treated 3 times weekly with a goal dosage of 4 times the initial dosage. Extra treatments to the extremities can be added at any time if deemed necessary. Maintenance therapy tends to be every 7–10 days to prevent relapse, and duration of maintenance therapy can range from months to years depending on the patient's disease course. Different equipment can change the required protocol and adjustments should be made according to patient's response and the clinician's judgment.

Cost

Starting a NB-UVB practice or adding to an existing one involves equipment costs, replacement parts, bulbs, staff training, etc. NB-UVB units with 48 bulbs cost USD 16,000–21,500. The best unit for a busy practice is one with the most bulbs in order to shorten light treatments. Additional considerations involve the need for standing platforms, built-in dosimetry and protocols, hand and foot units, hand-held units for localized areas, and units for the scalp with removable comb attachment. Home phototherapy units, including 4- to 6-foot phototherapy light panels with foldable wings, hand and foot units, and handheld units are available from the National Biological Corporation.

The following companies offer NB-UVB bulbs (TL-01 fluorescent lamps) of various sizes: National Biological Corporation, Daavlin, Phillips Company, and Psoralite Corporation. As energy output decreases with usage of the bulb, patients must remain in the light box for longer periods of time in order to receive the adequate dose. In a high-volume practice, it is more cost effective to replace bulbs promptly and maintain short patient visits. Measuring light output is also an important part of safe and effective phototherapy. National Biological Corporation machines are sold with built-in dosimetry meters so that output is machine-monitored and calibration needs to be done only once yearly.

Broadband UVB

BB-UVB with coal tar was used by William Goeckerman in the 1920s for moderate to severe psoriasis [27] (see 'Day treatment programs: Goeckerman therapy and Ingram therapy'). The application of coal tar combined with erythrogenic UV exposure to the skin can be highly effective. However, published literature on BB-UVB alone for the treatment of psoriasis remains limited.

Efficacy

The most effective wavelengths of UVB light used for the treatment of psoriasis fall in a very narrow range, 311–313 nm [3]. This has led to the development of NB-UVB phototherapy, which is more efficacious than broadband phototherapy as shown in multiple comparative studies [3–6]. Clearance is more rapid [3, 7], requires fewer treatments in some cases, and is preferred by more patients [5, 8]. This has explained the wide-spread transition within the last 20 years to NB-UVB for the treatment of psoriasis. BB-UVB (290–320 nm) continues to be used in the treatment of other dermatoses, such as atopic dermatitis, prurigo nodularis, pityriasis lichenoides chronica, uremic pruritus, and idiopathic pruritus.

Safety

Data on the incidence and severity of burning when compared to BB-UVB are controversial. Burning episodes with NB-UVB have been reported as fewer than [5, 7], equal to [4], and more [3, 8] than with BB-UVB. In patients treated for many years with conventional UVB, there is essentially no increased risk of skin cancer [17].

Dosage and Administration

Administration of BB-UVB is similar to that of NB-UVB. Initial dose can be determined by MED testing or by skin type as in NB-UVB. However, if dosage is to be determined by skin type, the starting dose is much lower for BB-UVB than for NB-UVB. Starting dose of BB-UVB for skin types are as follows (in mJ/cm^2): type I, 10; type II, 20; type III, 30; type IV, 40; type V, 50; type VI, 60. Increases in light on subsequent visits that occur within 3 days of the last visit are as follows (in mJ/cm^2): type I, 5; type II, 10; type III, 15; type IV, 25; type V, 25; type VI, 30. If visits occur later than 3 days after the last treatment, light should be increased more gradually than the above protocol, should not be increased at all, or, if a substantial amount of time has lapsed, decreased based on clinical judgment.

Psoralen plus UVA

PUVA uses a photosensitizing medication taken orally or absorbed topically in combination with UVA (320–400 nm) phototherapy. Treatment with UVA monotherapy produces only mild to moderate improvement, and is not recommended if other forms of phototherapy are available. PUVA penetrates more deeply into the tissue than UVB or NB-UVB, and is more effective than its UVB counterparts (especially for hand and foot psoriasis and eczema, due to the thicker skin involved in these anatomical locations); PUVA also provides a longer remission period than UVB. After 30 years of use, PUVA continues to be one of the best psoriasis treatments available, especially for recalcitrant or widespread cases of psoriasis.

Efficacy

There are several scenarios where PUVA therapy is preferred, including patients with a long history of psoriasis, thick plaques, and palmoplantar involvement. Furthermore, patients with nail involvement usually respond well to PUVA, with a 70% response rate after 3–4 months of treatments. Like UVB, PUVA requires a time commitment, at least initially, but can be tapered to a maintenance regimen as infrequent as once per month in patients who achieve a complete remission. This is in contrast to UVB and NB-UVB, where frequency of at least once a week is usually needed for effective maintenance. PUVA involves the use of psoralen (e.g. 8-methoxypsoralen, Oxsoralen Ultra®, ICN Pharmaceuticals, or 5-methoxypsoralen, Geralen®, Gerot Pharmazeutika) prior to exposure to UVA radiation. Improvement is usually seen after 6–10 treatments, followed by clearance of most lesions after 20–30 treatments [28].

It is well known that the systemic absorption of oral psoralen is associated with many risks, including the risk of developing cutaneous malignancies after long-term or high-dose therapy [29]. In order to reduce these side effects, bath PUVA was developed and has been associated with equal efficacy and fewer side effects, although being less convenient than oral PUVA is an obvious limitation. Soak PUVA is similar

a study of 80 patients with less than 10% BSA involvement receiving excimer laser therapy, 72% percent of patients achieved at least 75% clearing in an average of 6.2 treatments. Thirty-five percent of patients achieved 90% clearing in an average of 7.5 treatments. In a follow-up study, 55% of patients reported overall satisfaction with laser treatments.

Another study showed clearance in 85% of patients (n = 102) under a protocol in which dosage was determined by a standard MED of non-involved skin, while, in a comparable group (n = 40), clearance was shown in 84% of patients under a different protocol in which dosage was determined by MED of the involved skin. The second protocol was justified by the tendency of psoriatic lesions to withstand a higher dosimetry than normal skin. The second group on average required fewer treatments (7.07 treatments vs. 13 treatments) and a lower cumulative dose (6.25 vs. 11.25 J/cm^2) [43]. Studies such as these made it evident that dosage should be determined by the lesion and its induration rather than the MED of non-involved skin.

Previously, excimer laser therapy was considered a treatment for mild to moderate psoriasis, frequently used in patients with less than 10% BSA affected. However, the authors have experienced effective use in patients with up to 20% BSA affected. The XTRAC® Ultra (Photomedex; Montgomeryville, Pa., USA) has an average power of 1–2 W and the newer XTRAC Velocity is 300–400% more powerful than XTRAC Ultra, with faster delivery. This allows physicians to consider laser therapy for patients with 10–20% BSA involvement. In clinical practice, excimer laser can be used in combination with topical therapies to achieve more rapid results. When excimer laser was used in combination with PUVA (n = 272) there was no change in efficacy, but patients went into remission in half the treatment time and with half the cumulative UVA dosage as compared to PUVA alone [44]. Laser has also been proven to be effective in patients with palmoplantar psoriasis and scalp psoriasis [45, 46].

Safety

The most common side effects of the excimer laser include erythema, blistering and hyperpigmentation. These side effects are limited to localized areas in contrast to larger areas seen with full-body treatments using traditional phototherapy. Patients may use topical steroids to minimize such side effects. As of this writing, there have been 400,000 treatments of psoriasis with the XTRAC laser, and no reports of associated skin cancer.

Dosage and Administration

The XTRAC laser excimer machine delivers monochromatic light as a uniform square beam measuring 4 cm^2, which may be used in either paint or tile mode.

In paint mode, monochromatic light is delivered continuously as the handpiece is moved over the plaques; many physicians use the more rapid paint mode in clinical practice. In tile mode, the handpiece is held in place, a predetermined amount of UV light is given, and the handpiece is moved to an adjacent area. Tile mode is preferred in the research setting as it allows better standardization between operators and centers.

Administration of excimer laser therapy is conducted twice weekly, for a series of 10 treatments, to start. There should be a minimum of 48 hours between treatments. Patients are encouraged to comply with the schedule as closely as possible. Patients may see a response following just 4–6 treatment sessions, and some patients notice marked reduction in pruritus after 24 h. Treatment times vary depending on the number, size, and induration of the psoriatic plaques. The center of plaques tends to clear more rapidly than the outer boundary.

When determining the dosage for administration of laser phototherapy, there is a standard protocol card which is included with XTRAC laser machines (table 2). Historically, physicians were constrained to 1–3 times the minimal erythema dose, which based UV light dosage on healthy tissue. However, psoriatic tissue has a much higher tolerance for blistering and erythema as compared to non-involved tissue. The current standard protocol used for the Photomedex XTRAC Ultra and XTRAC Velocity machines is based on induration rather than MED, and uses the actual dose of light as measured in millijoules, rather than adjusting dosimetry by multiples of MED. This protocol also takes Fitzpatrick skin type into account, and was established by PhotoMedex by reviewing over 30 clinical trials. The PhotoMedex protocol included is simply used for illustration, and other excimer laser machines may have differing protocol regimens.

As patients are treated, psoriatic plaques become acclimatized to previous dosages and may require higher doses of light for further improvement [47]. Additionally, physicians must be careful to ensure that thinning lesions do not receive an excessively high dose such that it results in blistering or erythema, even though the same dose was tolerated previously when the plaques were thicker. The standard induration-based protocol, with incremental dosing changes, takes such factors into account. Another advantage in targeted UVB phototherapy is that different regions of the body can have differing optimal therapeutic doses of UV light, as higher doses can be targeted towards thicker plaques.

Cost

The current price for the XTRAC Ultra machine is USD 79,900; at the time of writing, the XTRAC Velocity price was to be announced.

Table 2. XTRAC Ultra and XTRAC Velocity excimer laser protocol

(A) Determining dose for first treatment of psoriasis

Plaque thickness	Induration score	Fitzpatrick skin type	
		FST 1–3 mJ/cm^2	FST 4–6 mJ/cm^2
Mild	1	300	400
Moderate	2	500	600
Severe	3	700	900

(B) Determining dose for subsequent treatments of psoriasis

Clinical observation				
No effect	Minimal effect	Good effect	Considerable improvement	Moderate/severe erythema
no erythema at 12–24 h, and no plaque improvement	slight erythema at 12–24 h, but no significant improvement	mild to moderate erythema response at 12–24 h	significant improvement with plaque thinning or reduced scaliness or pigmentation occurred	with or without blistering
Typical dosing change from prior treatment dose				
increase dose by 25%	increase dose by 15%	maintain dose	maintain dose or reduce dose by 15% (reduction intended to minimize hyperpigmentation effect and/or to avoid increased erythema)	reduce dose by 25% (treat around any blistered area; do not treat blistered area until healed with crust disappeared)

This dosing guideline is provided for guidance purposes only. Each patient may react differently; therefore, the physician should determine the actual treatment regimens based on patient history and their own clinical experience and expertise.
XTRAC Clinical Reference Guide: Dosing Guideline for Targeted UVB Phototherapy of Psoriasis. Ref: XTRAC Treatment Guidelines. 12-95359-01 Rev. C.

Combination Therapy

UVB and Topical Steroids

The effect of potent topical steroid cream used together with UVB phototherapy on clearing of psoriatic lesions as well as duration of remission was examined by Dover et al. [48]. A randomized double-blind placebo-controlled study was conducted with patients being treated with UVB, 3 times a week, with approximately half the patients applying topical corticosteroids twice daily and the other half applying placebo. The study found that there was no statistical significance in clearance rates. Furthermore, there were no statistically significant differences in the number of treatments or dosages of UVB required in order to achieve clearance. This study is in agreement with other earlier studies that also found there to be no advantageous effects of combination UVB and topical steroids, at least for traditional non-laser UVB phototherapy. However, from the authors' experience with localized recalcitrant plaques, topical therapy including super-potent topical steroids can significantly enhance UVB phototherapy. This is not surprising since it is easier to demonstrate enhanced benefit from combination therapy when dealing with more resistant plaques rather than plaques that are easier to eradicate.

PUVA and Topical Steroids

In contrast to studies with UVB, data regarding the use of topical steroids in combination with PUVA have shown some benefits. In a comparison of studies by Meola et al. [49], 5 studies examining PUVA alone versus PUVA with topical steroids showed more rapid rates of clearing and fewer quantitative UVA doses with the latter. However, 1 of the studies in the review did show a higher relapse rate with corticosteroid use [50].

Day Treatment Programs: Goeckerman Therapy and Ingram Therapy

Traditionally, day treatment programs can be classified into 2 main types: Goeckerman therapy, consisting of long skin contact with crude coal tar (CCT) combined with daily UVB light treatment, and Ingram therapy, consisting of the application of anthralin with UVB treatment, although both may be used simultaneously. While Goeckerman therapy is one of the oldest known treatments for psoriasis, it stands as one of the most effective as well. Day treatments were originally designed to minimize cost and maximize convenience for patients that required inpatient hospitalization, since patients with severe generalized psoriasis often require a treatment period of 4–6 weeks to clear their psoriasis completely. Day treatments are generally indicated for patients whose psoriasis is resistant to phototherapy or systemic agents, or for patients who are not eligible for systemic therapy. At the University of California San Francisco Psoriasis Center, patients typically receive phototherapy in the mornings and subsequently are coated with tar from the neck down. Skin is then occluded with saran wrap for 5–6 h. For patients that are applying tar for the first time, they should first receive a test dose of 2% CCT to 1 extremity for 1 day as tar may cause irritation to the skin. If tolerated, tar can be increased to 5% CCT and within several days to

10% CCT, if tolerated. If a patient proves to have a truly recalcitrant case of psoriasis, therapy can be escalated to combine anthralin, bath PUVA, acitretin or calcipotriene/tazarotene, as demonstrated in a study by Koo and Lee [51]. After 8 weeks of this regimen, 95% of 25 patients achieved PASI-75, and at 12 weeks 100% achieved PASI-75 [51]. Ingram therapy in combination with PUVA has been shown to clear subjects' lesions more readily than PUVA alone, but patients disliked the tendency of anthralin to temporarily stain the skin [50].

Motivated patients that have had previous experience in Goeckerman day treatments may self-administer Goeckerman therapy at home. Nightly applications of tar and/or anthralin with occlusion combined with phototherapy using home light boxes may prove to be a combination more convenient for patients who are unable to be admitted to the Day Center due to distance, jobs, etc.

Phototherapy and Systemic Retinoids

As a class, oral retinoids are not as efficacious as phototherapy or methotrexate [52]. However, in combination with UVB and PUVA, the effectiveness of acitretin for plaque-type psoriasis is markedly improved [53]. Combination with phototherapy may decrease the dose of both acitretin and phototherapy required for clinical improvement, while also maximizing efficacy and decreasing adverse effects.

Acitretin can be used to enhance PUVA or UVB phototherapy at a dosage ranging from 10 to 50 mg/day. Acitretin is especially useful for patients with extremely indurated and hyperkeratotic lesions in whom UVB radiation may not penetrate adequately unless the lesion is thinned by acitretin or a keratolytic agent such as 10% salicylic acid.

There are 2 approaches when using acitretin to enhance UVB phototherapy. The first is to start the patient on acitretin (typically 25 mg/day) approximately 2 weeks before starting phototherapy in order to prepare the skin for phototherapy. The second is to reserve low-dosage acitretin as a supplement after attempted UVB phototherapy alone proves unsatisfactory. However, adding low-dosage acitretin (25 mg/day or less) to established UVB phototherapy increases the possibility of developing delayed retinoid burn approximately 7–21 days after initiating acitretin. To minimize the risk of burning, it is important to decrease the intensity of UVB therapy by up to 50% approximately 7 days after initiating low-dosage acitretin supplementation. If no photosensitivity develops, UVB radiation can be gradually increased to previous levels.

Hydroxyurea

Hydroxyurea (Hydrea®) is another systemic agent that can be used to enhance UVB or PUVA phototherapy. The usual dosage is 500 mg orally twice daily. Like low-dosage acitretin, it is well suited for long-term enhancement of phototherapy in patients who experience a partial response to phototherapy alone. Hydroxyurea is not as effective as methotrexate. However, one of the main advantages of hydroxyurea when compared to methotrexate is the minimal risk of hepatotoxicity associated with its long-term use. Hydroxyurea can be an alternative for a patient who is a candidate for methotrexate, but refuses to undergo a liver biopsy. Another advantage is that hydroxyurea used to enhance UVB phototherapy does not increase the risk of photosensitivity, as seen with acitretin. However, hydroxyurea has a narrow therapeutic index, and can be associated with bone marrow suppression and nephrotoxicity.

Methotrexate

Methotrexate can be used in conjunction with UVB phototherapy. In 1982, Paul et al. [54] conducted a study examining methotrexate in combination with BB-UVB, while in the same year Morrison et al. [55] studied methotrexate in combination with PUVA [57, 58]. Both studies demonstrated that, when used in combination, the number of phototherapy sessions and the dose of BB-UVB or UVA could be reduced by more than half.

The following describes 3 approaches to using methotrexate in combination with phototherapy:

1 Methotrexate is used to control widespread inflammation in a patient presenting with intense erythroderma prior to starting UVB phototherapy. This is especially useful if the patient is not a candidate for cyclosporine or is unable to participate in day treatment.
2 Methotrexate is used in the short-term, while initiating UVB phototherapy, as an initial push to the therapeutic process.
3 Methotrexate is used to enhance phototherapy when a patient's response to UVB phototherapy plateaus, in a similar manner as acitretin and hydroxyurea are used to enhance phototherapy.

However, this combination should be used with extreme caution due to the rare risk of acute photosensitivity generally occurring within 48–72 h [54]. For example, a patient undergoing UVB phototherapy on Mondays, Wednesdays, and Fridays may start a weekly dose of methotrexate on Friday morning right after receiving phototherapy. By the time he or she returns for UVB phototherapy on Monday, the risk of methotrexate photosensitivity is negligible. By using this combination, one can minimize the cumulative methotrexate needed to clear the psoriasis. Once psoriasis clears completely, methotrexate can be discontinued altogether and patient's disease can usually be controlled with UVB phototherapy alone. Additionally, some patients are referred to outpatient UVB therapy or the day treatment program for the specific purpose of tapering off methotrexate after receiving a high cumulative dose. Of note, 1 small study suggests that treatment with methotrexate in combination with PUVA may increase the risk of squamous cell carcinomas [55].

Cyclosporine

The combination of cyclosporine and PUVA can increase the risk of skin cancer in Caucasian patients. Long-term use of cyclosporine with phototherapeutic modalities is not currently recommended [56]. However, there is one frequently encountered setting in which cyclosporine can be of great assistance in conducting phototherapy: erythrodermic patients. Erythrodermic patients have a high likelihood of exhibiting a paradoxical worsening reaction when receiving either PUVA or UVB. Therefore, the inflammatory state must be adequately controlled by means of a 'cool down' procedure that may consist of topical steroids, cool compresses, soothing baths, and more recently by short-term use of cyclosporine 3–5 mg/kg/day divided twice daily. When compared to methotrexate or acitretin for cooling down erythrodermic patients, cyclosporine has a faster onset of action. Once the inflammatory state has been controlled, phototherapy can be initiated very cautiously and the cyclosporine dosage tapered down to 3 mg/kg/day, and subsequently tapered down altogether once phototherapy has been optimized.

In a 2003 study, sequential therapy with cyclosporine and NB-UVB was compared to therapy with NB-UVB alone [57]. In this study, 30 patients with severe psoriasis received 3 mg/kg/day of cyclosporine for 4 weeks, followed by phototherapy with NB-UVB 3 times a week, while another 30 patients received NB-UVB monotherapy. Both treatment groups achieved marked improvements in their PASI scores, and treatment regimens were well tolerated in both study arms. However, in patients receiving 4 weeks of cyclosporine treatment, the number of NB-UVB exposures and cumulative dosage of UVB light was decreased.

Using cyclosporine for short periods of time (3 months or less) or at doses less than 5 mg/kg/day decreases the risk of nephrotoxicity. Moreover, the increased risk of malignancy can also be minimized by short-term use [56, 57]. Hypertension may be encountered, but is readily reversible with initiation of an antihypertensive agent or adjusting the dosage of cyclosporine.

Efalizumab

Combination therapy of NB-UVB with efalizumab (Raptiva®, Genetech, San Francisco, Calif., USA), a humanized monoclonal IgG1 antibody, was recently evaluated in an open-label single-arm clinical trial of 20 patients [58]. PASI-75 was achieved in 65% of patients at week 12. This result compares favorably to efalizumab monotherapy with a 22–27% PASI-75 response rate in randomized placebo-controlled phase 3 trials, and a 41% PASI-75 response rate in an open-label phase 3 trial [58]. No serious adverse events were reported in these patients receiving combination therapy. Efalizumab is being withdrawn from the market because of a potential risk to patients of developing progressive multifocal leukoencephalopathy (PML).

Alefacept (Amevive®)

Data for the combination of NB-UVB phototherapy and alefacept (Astellas Pharma, Tokyo, Japan) from a 12-week randomized split-body study of 14 subjects found that UV irradiation increased the mean PASI score by week 3; by week 12, PASI-75 was achieved in 86% of the irradiated body halves compared to only 43% of the control body halves, with complete remission occurring in 43% of UVB halves compare to none of the control sides [59]. This preliminary study provides promising evidence that combination therapy with NB-UVB may lead to clinically important increases in efficacy. NB- and BB-UVB therapy have been combined with alefacept in 2 center studies without an increase in skin cancer or other adverse events [60]. The combination of UVB phototherapy with alefacept resulted in a more rapid onset of response, and may be more efficacious than alefacept alone. There was no evidence of increased phototoxicity or photosensitivity with the combination. There are no reported data on the combination of alefacept with PUVA.

Etanercept

Recently, a multicenter open-label single-arm prospective study (the Utilization of NB-UVB Light Therapy and Etanercept for the Treatment of Psoriasis, UNITE, study) evaluated the efficacy of etanercept (Enbrel®; Amgen-Wyeth, Philadelphia, Pa., USA) 50 mg twice weekly in combination with NB-UVB 3 times weekly in patients with moderate to severe psoriasis (n = 86) [61]. After 12 weeks, the number of patients achieving PASI-75 response was 84.4%, as compared to 49% reported in etanercept monotherapy [62]. In this study, the combination of etanercept and NB-UVB was efficacious and generally well tolerated with no increase in photosensitivity noted. The addition of NB-UVB may serve as an option for the subset of patients who experience worsening of psoriasis after 'stepping-down' from the induction dose of 50 mg twice weekly to maintenance dose of 50 mg once weekly. Caution should be used when starting etanercept for patients with known or suspected skin cancers due to case reports of squamous cell carcinomas that grew rapidly from pre-existing suspicious lesions after initiation of etanercept therapy [63].

Summary

Despite many recent advancements in psoriasis treatment, phototherapy remains among the safest, most effective, and most versatile treatments for psoriasis. Nevertheless, the limitations of phototherapy need to be recognized. First and foremost, office phototherapy can be a major inconvenience. There is time spent in the office preparing for and undergoing the phototherapy treatment, and traffic and parking time needs to be included in the expected time lost from work. While day treatment programs may be extremely safe and effective, they are the least convenient way to manage psoriasis. For some patients, the inconvenience of phototherapy (and the cost as well) may be ameliorated through the use of home phototherapy. If office phototherapy is not available, tanning bed treatments may be beneficial for some patients [64]. As with all other forms of psoriasis therapy, it is essential to consider the impact of the treatment on the patient's lifestyle when selecting the treatment plan.

References

1 Parrish JA, Jaenicke KF: Action spectrum for phototherapy of psoriasis. J Invest Dermatol 1981;76:359–362.

2 van Weelden HE, Young E, van der Leun JC: Therapy of psoriasis: comparison of photochemotherapy and several variants of phototherapy. Br J Dermatol 1980;103:1–9.

3 Coven TR, Burack LH, Gilleaudeau R, Keogh M, Ozawa M, Krueger JG: Narrowband UV-B produces superior clinical and histopathological resolution of moderate-to-severe psoriasis in patients compared with broadband UV-B. Arch Dermatol 1997;133:1514–1522.

4 Karvonen J, Kokkonen EL, Ruotsalainen E: 311 nm UVB lamps in the treatment of psoriasis with the Ingram regimen. Acta Derm Venereol 1989;69:82–85.

5 Picot E, Meunier L, Picot-Debeze MC, Peyron JL, Meynadier J: Treatment of psoriasis with a 311-nm UVB lamp. Br J Dermatol 1992;127:509–512.

6 van Weelden H, De La Faille HB, Young E, van der Leun JC: A new development in UVB phototherapy of psoriasis. Br J Dermatol 1988;119:11–19.

7 Green C, Ferguson J, Lakshmipathi T, Johnson BE: 311 nm UVB phototherapy – an effective treatment for psoriasis. Br J Dermatol 1988;119:691–696.

8 Larkö O: Treatment of psoriasis with a new UVB-lamp. Acta Derm Venereol 1989;69:357–359.

9 Fischer T, Alsins J, Berne B: Ultraviolet-action spectrum and evaluation of ultraviolet lamps for psoriasis healing. Int J Dermatol 1984;23:633–637.

10 Hofer A, Fink-Puches R, Kerl H, Wolf P: Comparison of phototherapy with near vs. far erythemogenic doses of narrow-band ultraviolet B in patients with psoriasis. Br J Dermatol 1998;138:96–100.

11 Walters IB, Burack LH, Coven TR, Gilleaudeau P, Krueger JG: Suberythemogenic narrow-band UVB is markedly more effective than conventional UVB in treatment of psoriasis vulgaris. J Am Acad Dermatol 1999;40:893–900.

12 Yones SS, Palmer RA, Garibaldinos TT, Hawk JL: Randomized double-blind trial of the treatment of chronic plaque psoriasis: efficacy of psoralen-UV-A therapy vs narrowband UV-B therapy. Arch Dermatol 2006;142:836–842.

13 Gordon PM, Diffey BL, Matthews JN, Farr PM: A randomized comparison of narrow-band TL-01 phototherapy and PUVA photochemotherapy for psoriasis. J Am Acad Dermatol 1999;41:728–732.

14 Tanew A, Radakovic-Fijan S, Schemper M, Hönigsmann H: Narrowband UV-B phototherapy vs photochemotherapy in the treatment of chronic plaque-type psoriasis: a paired comparison study. Arch Dermatol 1999;135:519–524.

15 Calzavara-Pinton PG, Zane C, Candiago E, Facchetti F: Blisters on psoriatic lesions treated with TL-01 lamps. Dermatology 2000;200:115–119.

16 George SA, Ferguson J: Lesional blistering following narrow-band (TL-01) UVB phototherapy for psoriasis: a report of four cases. Br J Dermatol 1992;127:445–446.

17 Lee E, Koo J, Berger T: UVB phototherapy and skin cancer risk: a review of the literature. Int J Dermatol 2005;44:355–360.

18 Alderson MR, Clarke JA: Cancer incidence in patients with psoriasis. Br J Cancer 1983;47:857–859.

19 Larko O, Swanbeck G: Is UVB treatment of psoriasis safe? A study of extensively UVB-treated psoriasis patients compared with a matched control group. Acta Derm Venereol 1982;62:507–512.

20 Pittelkow MR, Perry HO, Muller SA, Maughan WZ, O'Brien PC: Skin cancer in patients with psoriasis treated with coal tar: a 25-year follow-up study. Arch Dermatol 1981;117:465–468.

21 Wulf HC, Hansen AB, Bech-Thomsen N: Differences in narrow-band ultraviolet B and broad-spectrum ultraviolet photocarcinogenesis in lightly pigmented hairless mice. Photodermatol Photoimmunol Photomed 1994;10:192–197.

22 Meola T, Soter NA, Ostreicher R, Sanchez M, Moy JA: The safety of UVB phototherapy in patients with HIV infection. J Am Acad Dermatol 1993;29:216–220.

23 Collins P, Ferguson J: Narrow-band UVB (TL-01) phototherapy: an effective preventative treatment for the photodermatoses. Br J Dermatol 1995;132: 956–963.

24 Belsito DV, Kechijian P: The role of tar in Goeckerman therapy. Arch Dermatol 1982;118:319–321.

25 Lowe NJ, Wortzman MS, Breeding J, Koudsi H, Taylor L: Coal tar phototherapy for psoriasis reevaluated: erythemogenic versus suberythemogenic ultraviolet with a tar extract in oil and crude coal tar. J Am Acad Dermatol 1983;8:781–789.

26 Shelk J, Morgan P: Narrow-band UVB: a practical approach. Dermatol Nurs 2000;12:407–411.

27 Perry HO, Soderstrom CW, Schulze RW: The Goeckerman treatment of psoriasis. Arch Dermatol 1968;98:178–182.

28 Melski JW, Tanenbaum L, Parrish JA, Fitzpatrick TB, Bleich HL: Oral methoxsalen photochemotherapy for the treatment of psoriasis: a cooperative clinical trial. J Invest Dermatol 1977;68:328–335.

29 Lebwohl M, Ali S: Treatment of psoriasis. 1. Topical therapy and phototherapy. J Am Acad Dermatol 2001;45:487–498, quiz 499–502.

30 Grundmann-Kollmann M, Tegeder I, Ochsendorf FR, Zollner TM, Ludwig R, Kaufmann R, Podda M: Kinetics and dose-response of photosensitivity in cream psoralen plus ultraviolet A photochemotherapy: comparative in vivo studies after topical application of three standard preparations. Br J Dermatol 2001;144:991–995.

31 Hannuksela-Svahn A, Sigurgeirsson B, Pukkala E, Lindelöf B, Berne B, Hannuksela M, Poikolainen K, Karvonen J: Trioxsalen bath PUVA did not increase the risk of squamous cell skin carcinoma and cutaneous malignant melanoma in a joint analysis of 944 Swedish and Finnish patients with psoriasis. Br J Dermatol 1999;141:497–501.

32 Lindelöf B, Sigurgeirsson B, Tegner E, Larkö O, Berne B: Comparison of the carcinogenic potential of trioxsalen bath PUVA and oral methoxsalen PUVA: a preliminary report. Arch Dermatol 1992; 128:1341–1344.

33 Stern RS, Nichols KT, Vakeva LH: Malignant melanoma in patients treated for psoriasis with methoxsalen (psoralen) and ultraviolet A radiation (PUVA): the PUVA follow-up study. N Engl J Med 1997; 336:1041–1045.

34 Lindelöf B, Sigurgeirsson B, Tegner E, Larkö O, Johannesson A, Berne B, Ljunggren B, Andersson T, Molin L, Nylander-Lundqvist E, Emtestam L: PUVA and cancer risk: the Swedish follow-up study. Br J Dermatol 1999;141:108–112.

35 Murase JE, Lee EE, Koo J: Effect of ethnicity on the risk of developing nonmelanoma skin cancer following long-term PUVA therapy. Int J Dermatol 2005;44:1016–1021.

36 Rapp SR, Parisi SA, Walsh DA: Psychological dysfunction and physical health among elderly medical inpatients. J Consult Clin Psychol 1988;56:851–855.

37 Asawanonda P, Anderson RR, Chang Y, Taylor CR: 308-nm excimer laser for the treatment of psoriasis: a dose-response study. Arch Dermatol 2000;136:619–624.

38 Bónis B, Kemény L, Dobozy A, Bor Z, Szabó G, Ignácz F: 308 nm UVB excimer laser for psoriasis. Lancet 1997;350:1522.

39 Kemény L, Bónis B, Dobozy A, Bor Z, Szabó G, Ignácz F: 308-nm excimer laser therapy for psoriasis. Arch Dermatol 2001;137:95–96.

40 Rodewald EJ, Housman TS, Mellen BG, Feldman SR: The efficacy of 308 nm laser treatment of psoriasis compared to historical controls. Dermatol Online J 2001;7:4.

41 Trehan M, Taylor CR: High-dose 308-nm excimer laser for the treatment of psoriasis. J Am Acad Dermatol 2002;46:732–737.

42 Feldman SR, Mellen BG, Housman TS, Fitzpatrick RE, Geronemus RG, Friedman PM, Vasily DB, Morison WL: Efficacy of the 308-nm excimer laser for treatment of psoriasis: results of a multicenter study. J Am Acad Dermatol 2002;46:900–906.

43 Gerber W, Arheilger B, Ha TA, Hermann J, Ockenfels HM: Ultraviolet B 308-nm excimer laser treatment of psoriasis: a new phototherapeutic approach. Br J Dermatol 2003;149:1250–1258.

44 Trott J, Gerber W, Hammes S, Ockenfels HM: The effectiveness of PUVA treatment in severe psoriasis is significantly increased by additional UV 308-nm excimer laser sessions. Eur J Dermatol 2008;18:55–60.

45 Nisticò SP, Saraceno R, Stefanescu S, Chimenti S: A 308-nm monochromatic excimer light in the treatment of palmoplantar psoriasis. J Eur Acad Dermatol Venereol 2006;20:523–526.

46 Morison WL, Atkinson DF, Werthman L: Effective treatment of scalp psoriasis using the excimer (308 nm) laser. Photodermatol Photoimmunol Photomed 2006;22:181–183.

47 Taneja A, Trehan M, Taylor CR: 308-nm excimer laser for the treatment of psoriasis: induration-based dosimetry. Arch Dermatol 2003;139:759–764.

48 Dover JS, McEvoy MT, Rosen CF, Arndt KA, Stern RS: Are topical corticosteroids useful in phototherapy for psoriasis? J Am Acad Dermatol 1989;20:748–754.

49 Meola T Jr, Soter NA, Lim HW: Are topical corticosteroids useful adjunctive therapy for the treatment of psoriasis with ultraviolet radiation? A review of the literature. Arch Dermatol 1991;127:1708–1713.

50 Morison WL, Parrish JA, Fitzpatrick TB: Controlled study of PUVA and adjunctive topical therapy in the management of psoriasis. Br J Dermatol 1978;98:125–132.

51 Lee E, Koo J: Modern modified 'ultra' Goeckerman therapy: a PASI assessment of a very effective therapy for psoriasis resistant to both prebiologic and biologic therapies. J Dermatolog Treat 2005;16:102–107.

52 Linden KG, Weinstein GD: Psoriasis: current perspectives with an emphasis on treatment. Am J Med 1999;107:595–605.

53 Tanew A, Guggenbichler A, Hönigsmann H, Geiger JM, Fritsch P: Photochemotherapy for severe psoriasis without or in combination with acitretin: a randomized, double-blind comparison study. J Am Acad Dermatol 1991;25:682–684.

54 Morison WL, Momtaz K, Parrish JA, Fitzpatrick TB: Combined methotrexate-PUVA therapy in the treatment of psoriasis. J Am Acad Dermatol 1982;6:46–51.

55 Fitzsimons CP, Long J, MacKie RM: Synergistic carcinogenic potential of methotrexate and PUVA in psoriasis. Lancet 1983;1:235–236.

56 Oxholm A, Thomsen K, Menne T: Squamous cell carcinomas in relation to cyclosporin therapy of non malignant skin disorders. Acta Derm Venereol 1989;69:89–90.

57 Krupp P, Monka C: Side-effect profile of cyclosporin A in patients treated for psoriasis. Br J Dermatol 1990;122(suppl 36):47–56.

58 Kircik LH, Liu Clive, Goffe BS: Treatment of moderate-to-severe plaque psoriasis with concomitant narrow-band UVB phototherapy and efalizumab: results from a multicenter investigator-sponsored trial. Presented at Summer Academy, Am Acad Dermatol, New York, August 2007, presentation P1805.

59 Legat FJ, Hofer A, Wackernagel A, Salmhofer W, Quehenberger F, Kerl H, Wolf P: Narrowband UV-B phototherapy, alefacept, and clearance of psoriasis. Arch Dermatol 2007;143:1016–1022.

60 Ortonne JP, Khemis A, Koo JY, Choi J: An open-label study of alefacept plus ultraviolet B light as combination therapy for chronic plaque psoriasis. J Eur Acad Dermatol Venereol 2005;19:556–563.

61 Kircik L, Bagel J, Korman N, Menter A, Elmets CA, Koo J, Yang YC, Chiou CF, Dann F, Stevens SR, Unite Study Group: Utilization of narrow-band ultraviolet light B therapy and etanercept for the treatment of psoriasis (UNITE): efficacy, safety, and patient-reported outcomes. J Drugs Dermatol 2008;7:245–253.

62 Papp KA, Tyring S, Lahfa M, Prinz J, Griffiths CE, Nakanishi AM, Zitnik R, van de Kerkhof PC, Melvin L, Etanercept Psoriasis Study Group: A global phase III randomized controlled trial of etanercept in psoriasis: safety, efficacy, and effect of dose reduction. Br J Dermatol 2005;152:1304–1312.

63 Smith KJ, Skelton HG: Rapid onset of cutaneous squamous cell carcinoma in patients with rheumatoid arthritis after starting tumor necrosis factor alpha receptor IgG1-Fc fusion complex therapy. J Am Acad Dermatol 2001;45:953–956.

64 Fleischer AB Jr, Clark AR, Rapp SR, Reboussin DM, Feldman SR: Commercial tanning bed treatment is an effective psoriasis treatment: results from an uncontrolled clinical trial. J Invest Dermatol 1997;109:170–174.

John Koo, MD
UCSF Psoriasis and Skin Treatment Center
515 Spruce Street
San Francisco, CA 94143 (USA)
Tel. +1 415 476 4701, Fax +1 415 502 4126, E-Mail john.koo@ucsfmedctr.org

Yawalkar N (ed): Management of Psoriasis.
Curr Probl Dermatol. Basel, Karger, 2009, vol 38, pp 79–94

Retinoids, Methotrexate and Cyclosporine

Louis Dubertret

Saint Louis Hospital, University Paris 7, Paris, France

Abstract

Acitretin alone is efficient (PASI 90: 40%). In responders, it is the best long-term maintenance treatment (up to 29 years of continuous treatment). The main side effect is its teratogenicity in females. It is necessary to begin retinoid treatment at low doses (10 mg/day), increasing the dose step by step, looking for the maximum well-tolerated dose (usually defined as a mild cheilitis). Doses higher than the highest well-tolerated dose are frequently responsible for the Köbner phenomenon. In children, retinoids are very efficient and nearly always well tolerated, but it seems important to never give more than 0.5 mg/kg/day. Methotrexate is the best treatment for severe psoriasis. Given at low doses once a week, it is a safe, cheap, convenient and efficient treatment, if carefully monitored. The main problem is the possible long-term liver toxicity of methotrexate. The risk is very low in patients not at risk (no liver disease). In these cases, liver biopsies are dangerous and useless. In the other cases, the need for liver biopsy is very rare, decided only by the hepatologist, and should be replaced by FibroTest and FibroScan. The old American guidelines should not be followed, and new guidelines are needed. Cyclosporine at low doses is an outstanding emergency treatment. It was first used as the last possible systemic treatment, but long-term continuous treatments are seldom possible due to alterations in kidney functions. A careful follow-up of kidney functions, with measurement of the glomerular filtration rate after each year of cumulative treatment, is necessary. The cyclosporine dose must be calculated according to the theoretical body weight in obese patients to avoid overdosage. Cyclosporine is mainly used now as a short-term treatment that is very efficient for young people, who find this illness particularly difficult. Cyclosporine is not contraindicated during pregnancy.

Acitretin, methotrexate and cyclosporine remain as the first-line systemic treatments of psoriasis, and their indications must be carefully evaluated for each patient before using biologicals for legal and safety reasons.

Retinoids

The antipsoriatic activity of aromatic retinoids (etretinate and its principal metabolite acitretin) was discovered by chance when these substances were being developed with the aim of producing anticancer agents. With varying affinity from one substance to another, retinoids bind to nuclear receptors (α-, β- and γ-RAR), though there is no way of currently establishing a correlation between the receptors involved and their antipsoriatic activity. It is known, however, that retinoids are capable of modifying the terminal differentiation of the epidermis. High doses are able to severely impair the skin barrier function of normal skin [1], but to improve terminal differentiation in psoriasis plaques [2]. They are also known to have strong anti-inflammatory activity, and more specifically are able to inhibit migration of the neutrophilic polynuclears from the capillaries of the superficial dermis towards the epidermis [3]. Finally, retinoids are capable of inhibiting antigen presentation by acting quite simultaneously on the Langerhans cells and T lymphocytes, though this immunosuppressive activity is far less than that of cyclosporine [4].

Aromatic retinoids are hydrophobic molecules (etretinate far more so than acitretin) that accumulate progressively in the adipose tissue. Their elimination is slow, the half-life being 120 days for etretinate and 2 days for acitretin. These 2 substances, like all retinoids, are powerfully teratogenic. In the presence of alcohol, it is possible to induce inverse metabolism and thus transform acitretin into etretinate, hence the need for 2 years' contraception after stopping treatment with acitretin as well as etretinate; 2 weeks are sufficient for ladies who have never drunk alcohol [5].

When psoriasis requires systemic treatment, acitretin and etretinate are the best long-term treatment, when efficient and well tolerated. Unfortunately, they are contraindicated in any woman contemplating motherhood, due to the need for contraception throughout the duration of the treatment and the 2 years following withdrawal.

The available retinoids are etretinate (Tigason®) and acitretin (Neotigason®/Soriatane®). Acitretin is the principal metabolite of etretinate. Etretinate and acitretin have the same therapeutic profile during the first months of treatment, but do not have the same side effects in the long term. Furthermore, some patients are more sensitive to one substance or the other. It is particularly detrimental, therefore, that these 2 substances are no longer available to patients in all countries.

The therapeutic effectiveness of retinoids shows up slowly, whereas their side effects for any given dosage appear within the first fortnight of the treatment. When the dose is reduced due to the side effects, they disappear within a fortnight of adjusting the dose. Therapeutic studies have shown that the maximum dose well tolerated by a patient is the most effective dose for that patient. In fact, with a high dose (0.5–1 mg/kg/day), the percentage of patients showing clearance (PASI 90%) was only 25%, whereas, when starting at a low dose (10 mg/day) and progressively increasing up to the maximum well-tolerated dose, the percentage of clear patients was 40% [Roche, unpublished report of a 1-year double-blind study].

Retinoids are thus the only family of drugs in the pharmacopoeia whose dosage is chosen not on the strength of their efficacy but on their tolerability, and hence the patient's quality of life. Effectively, the side effects are basically harmless, albeit highly uncomfortable at times due to the weakening of the epithelium and integumentary system brought about by these agents.

Prescription Strategy

The rules for prescription are particularly simple. Usually, start off on 10 mg/day with meals, then increase the doses by increments of 5 mg of the daily dose, either fortnightly or monthly, until the maximum tolerated dose is found, i.e. most commonly, the dose entailing tolerable cheilitis. If this dose is exceeded, have the patient reduce the dose until the maximum well-tolerated dose is again found [6–8]. Efficacy is judged by the improvement in the skin observed 3 months after reaching the maximum dose that is perfectly well tolerated.

It needs to be stressed that for each patient retinoid activity goes through 3 phases, according to dosage. At very weak doses, there is no therapeutic effect. Then, if it exists, the therapeutic efficacy dose is reached. If this dose is exceeded, the retinoids may weaken the skin to the point where aggravation of the psoriasis is caused by Köbner's phenomenon. The dose variation between inefficacy and intolerability may be as low as 5 mg. Given their long half-life, it is always possible to adjust treatment with retinoids in increments of 5 mg, varying the number of 10-mg tablets taken on even and uneven days, for example.

Side Effects

The side effects of retinoids are dose dependent [7]. However, the maximum well-tolerated dose is extremely variable from one patient to another, potentially ranging from less than 10 mg/day up to more than 75 mg/day. The reasons for these variations are not well understood, and are likely to couple sizable variations in retinoid absorption capacity with highly variable individual sensitivity to these drugs. This great variability explains why it is preferable to start off with very small doses, given that the drug is not prescribed for emergency situations. If this individual sensitivity cannot be predicted, it must be stressed that the weakening of the skin by the retinoids will increase with age and is often severe in atopic subjects.

The clinical side effects essentially result from a weakening of the epithelia and their products, nails and hair, by the retinoids. The earliest side effect is generally cheilitis. Dryness of the eyes is frequent and contact lenses are contraindicated. Rhinitis sicca, sometimes with epistaxis, is not uncommon. Fragility of the skin can be accompanied by pruritus, particularly in all rubbing or friction zones. Retinoids can frequently trigger (sometimes fierce) senile pruritus. At strong doses, retinoids generate hair cycle synchronization, with hair loss of sometimes spectacular proportions. Regrowth is usual on discontinuing the treatment, but may be incomplete. Conversely, retinoids may modify the texture of the hair, making it look more or less curly and sometimes unmanageable. Nail growth may be disturbed, sometimes producing Köbner's phenomenon at this level, entailing the development of ungual psoriasis, sometimes severe. The periungual skin may be weakened, promoting the development of granulation tissue, particularly on the feet.

Apart from such epithelial fragility, numerous other side effects may be observed: a reduction in night vision that may be dangerous in the case of long-distance lorry drivers, mood swings capable of leading up to depression and libido decrease, as well as a faster appearance of muscle aches contraindicating the use of retinoids in elite sportsmen and sportswomen. Headaches can be debilitating.

Numerous other side effects may be observed, which may be unpleasant but are quite harmless. The patient must be informed that in the event of any disturbing side effect ascribed to retinoids, the most simple solution is to stop the treatment for a fortnight; actually, there is no rebound phenomenon from discontinuing retinoids. If the trouble disappears and then reappears when the treatment is resumed, it is because it is connected with retinoids. On the basis of his/her quality of life and the therapeutic results, it is then up to the patient to choose whether or not to continue with retinoids.

The main side effect of retinoids is their teratogenicity. Provisions must be made for totally effective contraception throughout treatment and for the 2 years after halting treatment. In practice, this restriction prevents retinoids being prescribed to fertile women. What should be done in the event of an onset of pregnancy during the 2 years following discontinuation of the treatment? For virtually all patients, acitretin is completely eliminated 1 month after treatment stops, and is therefore no longer any teratogenic risk. To verify this, it is possible to determine the quantity of retinoids in the blood (e.g. by Roche Laboratories).

Biomonitoring

Biological monitoring (biomonitoring) is quite simple, as it will suffice to make a quantitative determination of transaminases, cholesterol and triglycerides before treatment, at the end of 1 month's treatment and then every 3 months. Acitretin more often increases triglycerides, whereas etretinate more often increases cholesterol. Lipid problems will be more frequent if the patient is obese, diabetic or abuses alcohol, and all of these situations are associated with hepatic steatosis. Only a large increase in triglycerides is a contraindication to starting treatment: in fact, acitretin may provoke a sudden increase in triglycerides in this case, with a risk of acute pancreatitis. There again, a moderate increase in triglycerides or cholesterol will simply provide an incentive to monitor the lipid balance every month and implement a diet. In the event of a progressive increase in cholesterol, the decision will be relative to the therapeutic improvement obtained: diet only, a lipid-lowering drug or discontinuation of retinoids.

Acitretin is only hepatotoxic in exceptional cases [9, 10], but may quite often bring about an increase in transaminases of 2 or 3 times the norm, particularly in patients with hepatic steatosis. In these situations, it is important to intensify biomonitoring (monthly monitoring), and to ask patients to cut out alcohol and excess sugar and fat. Prescribing polyunsaturated omega–3 fatty acids (MaxEPA®) seems to be able to improve this situation and reduce the cutaneous side effects of the retinoids. However, this has still to be demonstrated, and does not eliminate the need for dieting anyway. Cirrhosis or hepatitis C and B are not contraindications to retinoids, but an indication for monthly monitoring and a proper joint effort with the hepatologist.

Bone Monitoring

Bone monitoring is useful in 2 different contexts: in the child and in the adult. In the child, retinoids are remarkably effective, but must always be monitored in liaison with the general practitioner (GP) or pediatrician to make certain that there is no deterioration in the growth curve. In adults, the risk is calcification of the tendon insertions. The presence of hyperostosis is more common in psoriatics than in normal subjects, but in some subjects it is clear that retinoids may favor the development of (sometimes spectacular) hyperostosis. Given the rarity of this side effect, systematic monitoring would seem to offer a very poor cost/benefit ratio. Conversely, if painful areas appear (a calcaneal spur, for example), it seems fair to perform bone scintigraphy and X-rays targeting any areas of hyperfixation. In the event of hyperostosis, it is then possible to monitor its development every 2 or 3 years. The indication for subsequently stopping retinoids is highly controversial, and each case must be considered on its own according to the therapeutic benefits observed by the patient. Some patients presenting pain-free hyperostosis that is clearly linked to the treatment refuse to stop taking retinoids due to the therapeutic benefits observed.

A few patients have been on retinoids for more than 30 years now, raising the problem of potential side effects over a very long period. Vigilance remains the keyword for these patients. Some of them present atrophy of the dermis, although this is difficult to interpret as these patients also make occasional use of a little topical corticotherapy. These observations have led to a study conducted for over 5 years to investigate the occurrence of osteoporosis in subjects on retinoid therapy. During this time, no significant variation was observed [11]. For treatments over a very long time, it seems reasonable to perform bone densitometry every 5 years to verify that the latter falls within the norm relative to the patient's age.

Strong Doses

Retinoids can be given in strong doses of almost 1 mg/kg/day in 2 circumstances:
Pustular psoriasis. High doses are given over 7–10 days, and thereafter reduced to tolerated doses. In this indication, acitretin or etretinate may be replaced with 13-cis-

retinoic acid (Roaccutane) in fertile women wishing to contemplate pregnancy. In fact, the anti-inflammatory effect sought – inhibition of neutrophilic polynuclear migration – is the same with 13-cis retinoic acid as with acitretin, and contraception can be stopped 1 month after discontinuing the treatment.
Psoriatic rheumatism. High-dose retinoids, approaching 1 mg/kg/day, bring about a clear improvement in some two thirds of cases, the downside being substantial cutaneous or mucous side effects. Methotrexate's efficacy/side effect ratio is generally more favorable in this indication, where retinoids are rarely used [12].

Retinoids for Children

Retinoids are the best first-line systemic treatment for children.

Children must not be given retinoids at a dose higher than 0.5 mg/kg/day. More often than adults, children will sustain discreet cerebral edema with cephalalgia and irritability of a nature that should bring treatment to a halt, and be resumed at much weaker doses or even contraindicated.

Retinoids and Psoriasis Erythroderma

In psoriatic erythroderma, retinoids may be a good treatment, but only in very low doses (10 or a maximum of 20 mg/day). At higher doses, there is a risk of causing Köbner's with oozing erythroderma, which is capable of rapidly jeopardizing a good prognosis.

Retinoids and Psoriasis in HIV

Retinoids are usually quite effective for psoriasis occurring in HIV patients [13].

Combination Therapies

Retinoids combine successfully with all topical treatments, but do heighten the irritant nature of some (vitamin D derivatives and, of course, topical retinoids). They potentiate the effectiveness of phototherapy and are increasingly being used in tandem with broad-spectrum UVB, TL01 UVB and PUVA. They provide faster and more frequent (+15% excellent results) clearance of lesions. They can even be useful in patients resistant to retinoids alone, as they potentiate phototherapy by countering the photoprotective thickening of the stratum corneum caused by the latter [14]. They can be combined with methotrexate provided that weekly or bimonthly monitoring of liver enzymes is carried out [15]. The potential interest of combining them with cyclosporine has never been clearly assessed.

The combination acitretin/TNFα inhibitors is quite interesting [16].

Finally, the combination of retinoids and tetracyclines is contraindicated, as it entails a risk of cerebral edema.

Retinoids are the best maintenance therapy over a very long time for psoriasis of patients in whom they are efficacious [17]. Their efficacy peaks after 1 year of treatment, so it will often be necessary to combine them with some quick clearing therapy from the outset, thereby allowing the patient's state to improve more quickly.

Methotrexate

Methotrexate remains the benchmark therapy for severe psoriasis and/or psoriasis associated with peripheral articular involvement. It is the treatment that offers the best efficacy/tolerability/convenience/cost ratio for psoriasis.

Despite having been used in psoriasis for more than 40 years, the reasons for its effectiveness remain poorly understood. In fact, its antifolic effect (it is a structural analogue of folic acid, a powerful inhibitor of dihydrofolate reductase) is undoubtedly insufficient to explain its effectiveness at weak doses used just once a week. Methotrexate has many pharmacological properties, each of which may contribute to its antipsoriatic activity: cytokine inhibition (IL-1, IL-6, TNFα), inhibition of LTB_4, PGE_2, PAF and histamine production; inhibition of adhesion and of intratissular migration of macrophages and neutrophilic polynuclears; induction of apoptosis (programmed cell death) in phase-S cells; inactivation of activated T lymphocytes at weak doses. The main constraint on its use is its hepatic toxicity, which is clearly overestimated. It is a teratogenic drug that persists in the tissues for several weeks after stopping treatment. It is partly linked to plasma proteins, and its free form is the active one. It is eliminated through the kidneys.

Pretreatment Testing

The pretreatment testing is strictly structured: to start with, a general clinical examination and a biological checkup must be performed. This has to include a blood count, in order to ensure the absence of any hematological anomaly, and above all the absence of macrocytosis. A quantitative creatininemia analysis will be needed to ensure that there is no renal insufficiency, and liver enzymes must be checked for the absence of hepatopathy. A systematic investigation for hepatitis B and C seems useful. HIV testing could be proposed. Effective contraception must be prescribed before treatment that will last throughout the treatment and for the 3 months following its discontinuation, in men as well as in women.

Chest X-rays are frequently proposed, but the rational is poor [18].

Strategy for Use

Strategies for use are different in the north and in the south of European Union.

The first dose of methotrexate should be 5 mg, in order to detect any intolerability or idiosyncrasy, and then it should then be raised to a dose somewhere between 20 and 25 mg once a week on a precise day chosen along with the patient and noted on the prescription. In order to improve methotrexate tolerance, 5 mg of folic acid should be taken every evening, except the day on which methotrexate is taken [19]. Many strategies for the prescription of folic acid are used without comparative studies, but even with 5 mg folic acid the day after injection the tolerance seems improved. In order to avoid therapeutic error wherever possible and to start treatment under the best conditions for bioavailability and digestive tolerance, it is preferable to start treatment by intramuscular or subcutaneous injection for the first 6 months. Once sure that the patient is properly trained and treatment is effective, it will of course be far more convenient to switch from injections to tablets (Novatrex®/Rheumatrex®). The tablets are often taken in 3 parts over a week: that is, for example, on Friday evenings at 8 p.m., Saturday mornings at 8 a.m. and Saturday evenings at 8 p.m. It is quite possible to administer the weekly dose in 2 parts. Taking the weekly dose in 1 part decreases the absorption, increases the risk of digestive disturbances and of turning the treatment into a boring routine, thereby making compliance less strict. It is not uncommon to observe a relapse during the changeover from subcutaneous administration to taking tablets, the oral method often being less effective, certainly due to an initial hepatic passage and less favorable bioavailability.

With methotrexate, a number of drugs need to be avoided, and these must be listed on the prescription. These are antifolics such as Bactrim, sulfamides, sulfones, drugs that reduce renal elimination (like probenecid) or drugs that displace methotrexate from its plasma bonds (like strong doses of aspirin or non-steroidal anti-inflammatories). It is, of course, quite possible to start methotrexate treatment while patients are taking small doses of aspirin or non-steroidal anti-inflammatories for psoriatic arthritis, for instance.

Side Effects and Monitoring

The side effects are the occurrence of digestive disturbances during the 2 or 3 days following injection, and a feeling of a (sometimes incapacitating) fatigue during the same period. The occurrence of (sometimes severe) mucitis is particularly observable in the elderly or in patients with folate or vitamin B_{12} deficiencies. Taking folic acid (5 mg/day), except on the injection day, greatly reduces these side effects without decreasing therapeutic efficacy. The appearance of macrocytosis and its progressive aggravation should alert the medical professional to check for a folate deficiency or alcohol abuse, and to lower the doses. Pancytopenia mainly occurs during the first weeks of treatment [20]. Erosion of psoriatic plaques is also an early sign of toxicity [21]. In case of the appearance of hepatic cytolysis 3 times above the highest normal values, the treatment must be stopped and the advice of a hepatologist must be requested.

The immunosuppression caused by methotrexate is weak at the doses used in psoriasis treatment in the absence any other immunosuppressants, but vigilance is still called for.

Contraception is essential, of course, in fertile women during treatment and for 3 months following its discontinuation, due to this drug's teratogenic properties and its prolonged presence in tissues. The same duration of contraception is also advisable in men, as methotrexate reduces spermatogenesis. On the other hand, contrary to what used to be suggested, there seems to be no point in storing and preserving sperm before undergoing treatment because inhibition of spermatogenesis is reversible at antipsoriatic doses.

Methotrexate is not demonstrated as mutagenic, and is not considered contraindicated in a patient who has had cancer. However, this drug does contribute to reducing immune defenses, and rare cases of Epstein-Barr virus lymphomas have been described in psoriatics on methotrexate.

Biomonitoring is simple. A blood count every week for 2 months and then every month will suffice, along with a dose of transaminases every month. This biomonitoring must be conducted during the 2 days prior to taking methotrexate, as there is often a transient cytolysis, of no significance, during the days immediately following treatment.

The major problem is monitoring the liver. Cirrhosis may develop with biological liver tests showing normal results for a long time, and the liver biopsy puncture is an examination entailing non-negligible morbidity and mortality. The old guidelines were to perform a liver biopsy puncture every time a cumulative dose of 1.50 g of methotrexate had been exceeded. French hepatologists consider this strategy to be quite excessive and to cause patients to take needless risks. They also consider that there is no evidence to believe that methotrexate entails hepatic risks in patients who have no progressive hepatopathy and consume little alcohol. Finally, the scales used by anatomical pathologists (liver specialists) to measure hepatic fibrosis do not seem suitable for monitoring hepatic fibrosis on methotrexate, which explains without doubt the disparities observed in the literature concerning the rate of cirrhosis that ranges from 0 to 7.4%. It is important then to work with a team of hepatologists trained to monitor this drug. Finally, it should not be forgotten that the existence of hepatic fibrosis is more common in psoriatics than in non-psoriatics, without knowing with any certainty if such thing as a 'psoriatic liver disease' exists or if psoriatics tend to be consumers of alcohol more than non-psoriatics.

A series of follow-up studies extending up to 10 years have suggested that the risk of hepatic fibrosis occurring while on methotrexate is extremely faint, if not none, in patients whose serum type III procollagen rate (increased when there is collagen synthesis) is normal and remains normal when monitored systematically every 3 months [22]. It seems useful, therefore, to dose type III procollagen in patients on methotrexate every 3 months. A liver biopsy is useless in patients whose type III procollagen rate stays within normal limits.

Conversely, it must be remembered that the increase in type III procollagen is absolutely not specific to any hepatic involvement whatsoever, and that the only consequence of its increase is to eliminate an item of information that would have given the green light for abstaining from liver biopsy. There remains a need to carry out a wide-ranging study comparing patients on methotrexate who drink no alcohol whatsoever with others who drink occasionally, in order to find out whether or not total abstention from alcohol might help avoid hepatic biopsy puncture.

Fortunately, the association of a biological test (FibroTest) with a new non-invasive technique (FibroScan) allows a very sensitive evaluation of hepatic fibrosis and reduces the need for liver biopsies [23]. Using these tests every 3 years, we stopped performing liver biopsies 6 years ago.

The pulmonary toxicity of methotrexate crops up in 2 different contexts:

- The first is a hypersensitivity syndrome with 39–40°C fever, coughing, dyspnea, the appearance of major eosinophilia and of a non-systematized pulmonary infiltrate. Needless to say, treatment must be stopped urgently and never resumed. Systemic corticosteroid treatment can be necessary. This illness is exceptional.
- The second problem is that of pulmonary fibrosis while on methotrexate. Although being used for over 40 years in dermatology without this side effect ever being noted [18], our colleagues from rheumatology have remarked on the appearance of pulmonary fibrosis in some patients 2 or 3 years after starting methotrexate treatment of rheumatoid polyarthritis; in contrast, they never utilize liver biopsy punctures. This illustrates that the side effects of a drug are not the same according to the pathology treated. It should also prompt dermatologists to be heedful of dyspnea occurring in psoriatics, because even if this side effect is exceptional in the treatment of psoriasis, it nevertheless needs to be borne in mind.

Methotrexate osteopathy is very rare [24], and another piece of good news is that methotrexate reduces the incidence of death due to vascular diseases in patients suffering from psoriasis or rheumatoid arthritis [25].

Combination Therapies

Methotrexate may be combined with all topical treatments. If combined with phototherapy, methotrexate needs to be injected on the Friday evening following the last session in order to avoid photoactivation. Methotrexate is not a photosensitizer but is phototransformed into a highly photosensitizing photoproduct, [2,4-diamino-6-pteridinyl] carboxaldehyde [26]. Methotrexate may be combined with retinoids, provided there is tighter hepatic monitoring, and with cyclosporine in exceptional cases. It is commonly combined with infliximab in order to decrease the production of anti-infliximab antibodies.

Cyclosporine

The history of treating psoriasis with cyclosporine is particularly interesting. Cyclosporine was isolated from a fungus found in a sample of soil on a high plateau in southern Norway in 1969. At the time, the Sandoz laboratories were looking for new antibiotic substances. Cyclosporine proved to be a second-rate antibiotic; however, its weak toxicity provided an incentive to pursue pharmacological studies, and in 1972 the laboratory of J.F. Borel discovered its immunosuppressive properties. In 1978, the first organ transplant succeeded, thanks to cyclosporine, and in 1979 the substance's antipsoriatic powers were fortuitously recorded in patients suffering from psoriasis arthritis.

The use of cyclosporine in psoriasis developed in 2 stages, 12 years apart. First, cyclosporine was used in patients resistant to all other treatments. Under these conditions, it was a last-resort treatment administered over a long period of time; in particular, beyond the first year of treatment, it was usual to observe a reduction in glomerular filtration often signaled, though not always, by an increase in creatininemia. This renal insufficiency, the upshot of irreversible renal fibrosis, left no choice but to stop the treatment once and for all. A second side effect, not always reversible after stopping treatment, was the appearance of hypertension, a frequent cause of halting the treatment. These 2 side effects, potentially serious and not completely reversible once the treatment stopped, initially prompted dermatologists to cut down on the indications for this drug, as it could only resolve particularly difficult situations for a limited time [27].

Twelve years after cyclosporine had started to be used in psoriasis, it was suggested using cyclosporine as a systemic treatment of first intention, but during short interventions so as to try avoiding renal toxicity and hypertension. It was then ascertained that these short interventions, nearly always very well tolerated, could bring about prolonged remissions in some 30% of patients. Today, cyclosporine has thus become a treatment of first intention, usually reserved for short interventions. This 3- or 4-month prescription is designed to cope with urgent situations or seasonal psychological intolerance to the illness. Though particularly appealing to sufferers, it remains to be proved that this new strategy will help avoid cumulative kidney toxicity [28].

Pretreatment Checkup

The pre-cyclosporine therapy checkup is quite standardized. It calls for:

- a complete clinical examination to make sure that there is no progressive disease;
- a complete blood count and an inflammation test to check that there is no major biological anomaly;
- creatininemia determination 3 days in a row to calculate the average creatininemia that will enable treatment dosage to be adjusted in relation to renal tolerability;

- monitoring of lipid levels, as cyclosporine can induce hypertriglyceridemia during the initial months of treatment [29];
- a gynecological checkup in women to ensure the absence of any papilloma virus lesion of the cervix; HPV proliferation might be aggravated by the immunosuppression produced by the cyclosporine;
- a dental examination to verify the absence of parodontopathy, which must be treated prior to treatment in order to reduce the risk of gingival hypertrophy triggered by the cyclosporine;
- finally, one must check for the absence of chronic viral diseases, hepatitis C and B or HIV, and also that the patient has not had strong doses of PUVA, which would contraindicate cyclosporine.

Tolerance to the treatment may be partly predicted beforehand, given that treatment cessation due to side effects is more frequent with advancing age, patient obesity, diastolic pressure bordering on the norm and average creatininemia close to the upper limits of the norm. One major advantage of cyclosporine is that it requires no contraception for women and all pregnancies on cyclosporine have completed without fetal problems. The ideal profile for benefiting from cyclosporine is therefore that of a young slim hypotensive woman.

Monitoring

Monitoring is simple:

- Creatininemia has to be determined every month (mornings, on an empty stomach and with no previous muscular exertion). If the creatininemia increases by more than 30% by comparison with the patient's base value and is not within the norm, we must then check the dosage – which is highly variable – and, if the increase is confirmed, lower the cyclosporine dosage.
- Arterial pressure must be measured every month.
- Triglycerides must be monitored every month for the first 3 months of treatment.
- The gynecological examination must be repeated every year for women.
- Whenever the cumulative duration of cyclosporine treatment has reached 1 year, a measurement of the glomerular filtration rate must be performed. This will provide a complete sense of security when it comes to renal tolerability. This is an inexpensive and non-invasive examination.

Side Effects

The main side effects, around which all clinical and biological monitoring are arranged, are nephrotoxicity and hypertension [27]. Moreover, these are the 2 prime causes of discontinuing cyclosporine. It must be remembered here that renal insufficiency brought about by cyclosporine may appear eventhough creatininemia remains in normal range. That is why regular renal functional explorations are necessary when monitoring this treatment. Hypertension brought about by cyclosporine is more frequent when diastolic pressure is high before treatment. It is not always reversible. In the event of hypertension appearing while on cyclosporine, a salt-free diet must be started; if that is not sufficient, one must then resort to calcium inhibitors. Of these, it is necessary to avoid Nifedipine (Adalat®), which promotes gingival hyperplasia, and give preference to the family of dihydropyrimidines, like nicardipine (Loxen®). If the latter are not effective, cyclosporine will have to be stopped. Side effects leading to the discontinuation of treatment increase with the duration of treatment, with the age of the patients, with base creatininemia, with increased pretreatment diastolic pressure and, undoubtedly, with the presence of obesity.

Other less severe side effects are observed with cyclosporine: an increase in facial hairiness (reversible on discontinuation of treatment) and a slight increase in skin infections (folliculitis, verrucas, herpes and shingles). The only cancers to increase in incidence under cyclosporine are the cutaneous squamous cells carcinomas, especially in patients who have had many PUVA sessions and more than 2 years of cyclosporine treatment [30]. No increase has been noted in the incidence of lymphomas, but this eventuality remains possible. Epstein-Barr virus lymphomas have been caused by the combination of cyclosporine and systemic corticotherapy.

Other side effects are gastrointestinal disturbances, gingival hyperplasia, the appearance of paresthesia at the beginning of treatment, fatigue, headaches and, exceptionally, convulsions. Finally, cyclosporine reduces the absorption of calcium and vitamin D_3.

Strategy for Use

Cyclosporine treatment is started at a dose somewhere between 2 and 3 mg/kg/day [for an overview, see 31]. The maximum dose prescribed in psoriasis is 5 mg/kg/day. At the very outset of cyclosporine use in psoriasis treatment, it has been suggested starting therapy at high doses (5 mg/kg/day), clearing the patient rapidly, then progressively reducing doses until a relapse is observed, in order to find the effective minimum dose. This strategy was very soon dropped, as it was more aggressive to the kidneys and, above all, less well received by the patient. In fact, the patient experiences a rapid alleviation combined with a psychological questioning associated to the sudden disappearance of a chronic illness, and then he witnesses the disease relapse with equivalent unrest. The strategy that has won acceptance is to start off with small doses in order to obtain progressive improvement in the illness, while keeping as a fallback (should this improvement be insufficient) the possibility of progressively increasing the cyclosporine doses without ever exceeding 5 mg/kg/day. The patient then benefits from a progressive improvement in his quality of life until the dose is found that will restore to him a satisfying quality of life, even if it does not achieve complete clearance. Even with this strategy, however, the number of patients who have to break off cyclosporine treatment due to its side effects increases with time, and after 5 years of treatment there are only about 5% of patients who are able to continue without complications.

The association of magnesium (100 mg/day) to cyclosporine seems able to protect the kidneys, but this remains to be proved.

In order to avoid overdosage in obese patients, the daily dose of cyclosporine must be calculated using to the theoretical weight (according to the body size) [32].

Due to its renal toxicity in prolonged therapy, it was suggested to use cyclosporine for a short intervention of 3–5 months, either as an emergency treatment or 'to turn a corner', or as a short-term clearing treatment prescribed in conjunction with a long-term slow-acting maintenance treatment (e.g. acitretin); thus, giving this last one time to act. Some patients use cyclosporine for 4–5 months every year, for example, in order to spend the summer enjoying normal social life.

This new therapeutic approach has led to cyclosporine being put forward as a systemic treatment of first intention. In these conditions, it has been observed that 30% of patients remained clear for 6 months after breaking off a short course of cyclosporine [28]. In order to increase the chances of obtaining prolonged remission, it is important not to stop cyclosporine suddenly, but to decrease doses gradually over 2 months. These observations have profoundly changed the way this drug is used. It is now suggested as a systemic treatment of first intention for young subjects in order to perform short interventions not exceeding 4 months, followed by 2 months of dose reductions.

The change in the pharmacokinetics of cyclosporine brought about by other drugs is so frequent that it is important for psoriatics being treated with it to report always this treatment to their GP, so that if a prescription is needed for some other disorder, the GP can bear the drug interactions in mind.

Combination Therapies

In order to potentiate the effects of cyclosporine, topical treatments (especially vitamin D derivatives) seem particularly interesting. Combining with phototherapy is contraindicated, due to the immunosuppressant role of cyclosporine, which may favor the development of squamous cells carcinomas. The sudden appearance of multiple squamous cells carcinomas has been observed in some patients on cyclosporine who had had high cumulative doses of PUVA therapy, sometimes a great number of years before the cyclosporine treatment. Intensive and prolonged PUVA therapy therefore contraindicates the use of cyclosporine. Cyclosporine may be combined with retinoids, though the potential interest of this combination has not yet been validated. The most interesting strategy is, without doubt, the use of retinoids as a relay of cyclosporine to reduce the speed and intensity of a relapse on cessation of this potent therapy. At weak doses, the cyclosporine/methotrexate combination is effective, but used exceptionally as no test is available to measure the importance of the immuno-suppression produced by combining these 2 treatments.

References

1 Elias PM, Fritsch PO, Lampe M, et al: Retinoid effects on epidermal structure, differentiation, and permeability. Lab Invest 1981;454:531–540.

2 Gottlieb S, Hayes E, Gilleaudeau P, et al: Cellular actions of etretinate in psoriasis: enhanced epidermal differentiation and reduced cell-mediated inflammation are unexpected outcomes. J Cutan Pathol 1996; 23:404–418.

3 Dubertret L, Lebreton C, Touraine R: Inhibition of neutrophil migration by etretinate and its main metabolite. Br J Dermatol 1982;107:681–685.

4 Dupuy P, Bagot M, Heslan M, et al: Synthetic retinoids inhibit the antigen presenting properties of epidermal cells in vitro. J Invest Dermatol 1989;93: 455–459.

5 Gronhoj Larsen F, Steinkjer B, Jakobsen P: Acitretin is converted to etretinate only during concomitant alcohol intake. Br J Dermatol 2001;145:1028–1029.

6 Dubertret L: Etretinate (Tigason, Europe; Tegisonn, USA) in psoriasis: advantages of low doses progressively increased. J Am Acad Dermatol 1985;13(part 1): 830–831.

7 Berbis P, Geiger JM, Vaisse C, Rognin C, et al: Benefit of progressively increasing doses during the initial treatment with acitretin in psoriasis. Dermatologica 1989;178:88–92.

8 Pearce DJ, Klinger S, Ziel KK, et al: Low-dose acitretin is associated with fewer adverse events than high-dose acitretin in the treatment of psoriasis. Arch Dermatol 2006;142:1000–1004.

9 Roenigk HH Jr, Callen JP, Guzzo CA, et al: Effects of acitretin on the liver. J Am Acad Dermatol. 1999;41: 584–588.

10 Weiss VC, Layden T, Spinowitz A, et al: Chronic active hepatitis associated with etretinate therapy. Br J Dermatol 1985;112:591–597.

11 Halverstam CP, Zeichner J, Lebwohl M: Lack of significant skeletal changes after long-term, low-dose retinoid therapy: case report and review of the literature. J Cutan Med Surg 2006;10:291–299.

12 Klinkhoff AV, Gertner E, Chalmers A, et al: Pilot study of etretinate in psoriatic arthritis. J Rheumatol 1989;16:789–791.

13 Buccheri L, Katchen BR, Karter AJ, et al: Acitretin therapy is effective for psoriasis associated with human immunodeficiency virus infection. Arch Dermatol 1997;133: 711–715.

14 Lebwohl M, Drake L, Menter A, et al: Consensus conference: acitretin in combination with UVB or PUVA in the treatment of psoriasis. J Am Acad Dermatol 2001;45:544–553.

15 Lowenthal KE, Horn PJ, Kalb RE: Concurrent use of methotrexate and acitretin revisited. J Dermatolog Treat 2008;19:22–26.

16 Gisondi P, Del Giglio M, Cotena C, et al: Combining etanercept and acitretin in the therapy of chronic plaque psoriasis: a 24-week, randomized, controlled, investigator-blinded pilot trial. Br J Dermatol 2008; 158:1345–1349.

17 Stern RS, Fitzgerald E, Ellis CN, et al: The safety of etretinate as long-term therapy for psoriasis: results of the etretinate follow-up study. J Am Acad Dermatol 1995;33:44–52.

18 Belzunegui J, Intxausti JJ, De Dios JR, et al. Absence of pulmonary fibrosis in patients with psoriasic arthritis treated with weekly low-dose methotrexate. Clin Exp Rheumatol 2001;19:727–730.

19 Salim A, Tan E, Ilchyshyn A, et al: Folic acid supplementation during treatment of psoriasis with methotrexate: a randomized, double-blind, placebo-controlled trial. Br J Dermatol 2006;154:1169–1174.

20 Al-Awadhi A, Dale P, McKendry RJ: Pancytopenia associated with low dose methotrexate therapy: a regional survey. J Rheumatol 1993;20:1121–1125.

21 Pearce HP, Wilson BB: Erosion of psoriatic plaques: an early sign of methotrexate toxicity. J Am Acad Dermatol. 1996;35:835–838.

22 Maurice PD, Maddow AJ, Green CA, et al: Monitoring patients on methotrexate: hepatic fibrosis not seen in patients with normal serum assays of aminoterminal peptide of type III procollagen. Br J Dermatol 2005;152:451–458.

23 Berends MA, Snoek J, de Jong EM, et al: Biochemical and biophysical assessment of MTX-induced liver fibrosis in psoriasis patients: FibroTest predicts the presence and FibroScan predicts the absence of significant liver fibrosis. Liver Int 2007;27:639–645.

all therapeutic interventions require some degree of monitoring to assure appropriate use and outcomes. Since efalizumab is self-administered, a greater onus is placed upon patients to remain compliant and initiate action in the face of potential adverse events. Hence, periodic monitoring primarily serves to remind, update, and educate patients regarding their disease and its treatment.

A monoclonal antibody targeting CD11a, efalizumab is indicated for the treatment of chronic plaque psoriasis. Off-label use includes atopic dermatitis, psoriasis limited to hands or feet, and discoid lupus erythematosus [5]. Regardless of the indication, efalizumab is administered subcutaneously, with the majority of patients able to reconstitute and self-inject efalizumab after a single training session [6].

Monitoring decision points fall into 3 categories: (1) known short-term drug-associated events; (2) known requirements for intervention and monitoring during intermediate and long-term therapy; (3) potential, sporadic events occurring anytime during therapy. At each monitoring point, there are several decisions to be made, not the least of which is whether a therapy continues to be appropriate for a given patient. These decisions are made based upon facts, experience, and prudent practice. At times, the decision points, facts, experience, or prudence may conflict. Such is the art of medicine.

In this summary, I propose monitoring decision points. At each time point, there are recommended assessments. The drug label or product monograph suggests some assessments, some recommendations are based upon experience, and yet other recommendations are based upon prudent medical practice. These recommendations should be considered a framework upon which to devise clinician- and patient-specific monitoring regimens.

Mechanism of Action

LFA-1 is a ligand comprised of 2 subunits: CD11a and CD18. LFA-1, expressed on T cells, B cells, macrophages, and neutrophils, interacts with ICAM-1 [7]. Leukocytes and endothelial cells express the adhesion molecule ICAM-1 [8], as do keratinocytes [9]. The cellular expressions of the ligand LFA-1 and its corresponding receptor (ICAM-1) anticipate the potential immunological activities of LFA-1/ICAM-1 interactions: namely, interactions between lymphocytes, antigen-presenting cells, endothelial cells, and keratinocytes.

Though the predominant mechanism impacting psoriasis is unknown, certain of the known immunological effects of efalizumab anticipated recognized treatment management challenges.

Studies: Label versus Practical

Labels are deliberated documents providing guidance for drug use. Each regulatory body evaluates clinical trial and post-marketing data to determine appropriate use, dosing, and precautions that apply to specific indications and defined dosing regimens. Medications developed within the past 10 years often have monitoring guidance as part of the label. More often than not, prudence and experience in clinical practice exceed monitoring suggestions provided in official drug labels. Biologics generally fall in the later category.

Monitoring

The easiest, least controversial, and most readily dealt with adverse events are those experienced by 30% of patients following the first administration and 15% following the second administration of efalizumab: mild constitutional symptoms and fever [10]. The decision to utilize a conditioning dose of 0.7 mg/kg followed the first phase I study and a subsequent phase II study, where related adverse events (fever/chills, myalgia, nausea, and vomiting) occurred as dose-related side effects [11]. Prior to and at the time of training a patient on self-administration of a drug, appropriate warnings and precautions should be given. For the most part, these subacute adverse events occur within a few hours of drug administration, are generally mild, and resolve within 4–8 h. Occasionally patients may require acetaminophen or ibuprofen to alleviate symptoms. In my practice and during the clinical trials, less than 1% of patients experience severer symptoms (generally headache), which may persist for several hours and may recur 1 or 2 injections beyond the second treatment.

The only consistent laboratory abnormality seen in patients receiving efalizumab is elevated circulating lymphocyte counts. Circulating lymphocytes counts are elevated in most patients within the first 3 weeks of commencing therapy. These counts generally remain below the upper limit of normal, and are generally sustained throughout the course of therapy. Patients may develop sporadic, and occasionally sustained, marked elevations of lymphocyte counts. There are no clinical consequences resulting from the lymphocytosis. To minimize confusion, laboratory personnel should be apprised of patients being treated with efalizumab.

Eight cases of thrombocytopenia were reported during the phase III clinical studies, while other cases are reported in the post-marketing experience. The 8 cases reported in the clinical studies are the best characterized. Two of the 8 cases were associated with clinically significant bleeding. All cases reversed upon discontinuation of efalizumab, and some were treated with systemic corticosteroids. The association between efalizumab and thrombocytopenia remains uncertain. Antiplatelet antibodies were requested in a minority of cases, leaving open the question as to whether the thrombocytopenia is a direct drug effect, immunologically mediated but modulated by efalizumab, or a coincident event. Nonetheless, the product monograph suggests monitoring platelets prior to initiating therapy, monthly for the first 3 months of therapy, and every 3 months there after [12]. Based upon the calculated incidence of thrombocytopenia, <0.0001, repeated laboratory tests appear to be of modest benefit even though inexpensive.

Flare and rebound are 2 elements tied but not unique to efalizumab. During the clinical studies, a small number of patients experienced flare of psoriasis, defined as worsening of psoriasis while on therapy. Consistent and meaningful definitions of have been attempted, but their utility and validity remain unconfirmed. Members of the medical board of the US National Psoriasis Foundation recommend a definition of rebound: increase in PASI of 150% compared to baseline or appearance of atypical and inflammatory morphological forms of psoriasis within 12 weeks of discontinuation of treatment [13]. The European Medicines Agency has modified the definition to suggest 8 instead of 12 weeks [14]. Both definitions fail to recognize the biological and clinical half-life of therapies, rendering the definitions of marginal applicability. Reportedly, 5% of patients reported rebound of psoriasis upon discontinuing treatment [15]. The majority of these patients were considered nonresponders, having achieved less than 50% improvement in psoriasis after 12 weeks of therapy.

Three points regarding flare and rebound are evident and corroborated by clinical experience. Many of those patients who subsequently develop a flare, develop a widespread inflammatory eruption of papules or small plaques within the first few weeks of therapy. There are few such patients. Rebound is most common in patients who fail to achieve at least a 50% improvement in PASI by 12 weeks of therapy and then abruptly discontinue treatment. Though efalizumab is believed to be associated with dramatic cases of flare and rebound, all therapies have to a greater or lesser degree patients in whom flare or rebound or both have occurred.

New or recurrent signs and symptoms of arthropathy remain contentious. Efalizumab has not shown significant efficacy in the treatment of psoriatic arthritis. Clinical experience suggests that some patients with psoriatic arthritis benefit with efalizumab therapy. Evaluation of arthritis and arthropathy reports in clinical studies has shown no clear difference between patients on efalizumab and those receiving placebo, regardless of the clinical history [16]. Yet there is no doubt that patients uncommonly experience an atypical tenosynovitis-like arthropathy: tender and painful forearms often associated with painful acral joints. The arthropathy may be isolated, symmetric, or asymmetric. Arthropathy may occur during therapy or soon after discontinuation and may correlate with flare or rebound. The arthropathy, even in severe instances, appears to be self-limiting.

Unlike TNF antagonists, there is no evidence that efalizumab impacts the infectivity or reactivation of *Mycobacterium tuberculosis* [12]. While some routinely evaluate all patients considering treatment with biologics, there are other considerations suggesting the contrary. Not the least of these considerations is the need to institute therapy for latent infection should a screening test return positive. Given the risk of drug-induced hepatitis using standard treatment of latent disease, and given the extremely low probability of active tuberculosis (TB) when treating with efalizumab, the risk-benefit profile favors not screening. Even with the argument that patients may be later switched to another treatment, a TNF antagonist, the same standards would dictate retesting for TB to capture those who were subsequently exposed to tuberculosis bacteria, particularly in regions where TB is endemic.

After the first 6 months of therapy, there appear to be no consistently reported adverse events. Sporadic infections, malignancies, and organ-specific disorders occur at rates similar to those in the general population [17–20].

I have observed instances of worsening psoriasis during therapy (flare) and rapid worsening of psoriasis after discontinuation of therapy (rebound) with every therapy I have used to treat psoriasis. Though during the clinical studies, efalizumab, with 5% of patients experiencing flare or rebound, was the champion [19]. Better patient selection and possibly better appreciation of the early signs of flare and rebound have reduced both phenomena in my practice to negligible. Attempts to quantify and evaluate interventions for flare and rebound provided modest guidance [15, 21]. A paradigm, initially sketched on paper in the back of an empty ball room by Alan Menter and myself and later improved with comments by others, provided the real crux of management [22]. I now approach patients with stable plaque psoriasis (no recent history of worsening, stable minor psoriatic arthritis, and red but not scarlet patches or plaques) without reservation. Those with inflammatory robust progression or unstable plaque psoriasis will often respond well to modest doses of cyclosporine, which then permits the introduction of efalizumab after 1 or 2 weeks of therapy. A few papules erupting on the trunk or about the folds are to be expected. If the eruption persists or becomes more problematic, a short course of modestly dosed cyclosporine may be necessary. Similarly, when discontinuing efalizumab, patients are made aware that should there be rapid advances or many inflammatory papules developing over a short time; cyclosporine for 2–6 weeks may be required. One key point is the use of brand Neoral. Generic cyclosporines do not appear to have the same pharmacokinetic properties as the brand cyclosporines. Generics are less effective, require higher doses, and are often less well tolerated than Neoral. I have not found methotrexate, systemic retinoids, or phototherapy to be effective in ameliorating the flares or rebounds. If the flare or rebound becomes well established, I have found no truly effective therapy. Nonetheless, nearly all patients, even those with severe exacerbations, resolve within 8 weeks of onset. With modest early monitoring, prudent patient selection and management, the frequency of the bothersome flares and rebounds can be reduced to below 1%. Interestingly, prior flare or rebound do not appear to be correlated with recurrence on re-exposure.

A final question: under what circumstances should therapy with efalizumab be interrupted or discontinued? As a matter of medical prudence, a patient diagnosed with a serious infection or malignancy should discontinue treatment. There is no data to provide guidance, but patients with non-melanoma cutaneous malignancies, cervix carcinoma in situ, and other typically non-invasive malignancies should be considered on a case-by-case basis. It may be advised to discontinue efalizumab a few weeks prior to invasive elective surgery: data in support of this recommendation is lacking. Efalizumab does suppress primary activation of T cells very well, and will therefore blunt the immunological response to vaccines. Because of the blunted response, administration of vaccines in the face of treatment with efalizumab is ineffective rather than unsafe. It is advised to discontinue efalizumab 4–6 weeks prior to administration of a required vaccine and recommence therapy 4 weeks after administration. As a measure of medical prudence, patients who are to be treated with efalizumab should have their vaccination requirements completed 4 weeks prior to beginning therapy. The previously stated information is based upon a measured response to neoantigen phi-X174 [23]. Recent results evaluating the immunological response to polyvalent vaccinations in patients receiving efalizumab suggest a blunted but acceptable immunological response, thereby bringing into question the need to discontinue efalizumab when vaccinating [24].

Summary

Efalizumab is demonstrably safe and effective in the treatment of moderate-to-severe, chronic plaque psoriasis. The mode of action, data from clinical studies, and postmarketing observations suggests that efalizumab is not associated with activation of latent tuberculosis and is not associated with increased rates or severity of primary tuberculosis infections. Early events (flare, rebound, thrombocytopenia, arthropathy), though uncommon, suggest CBC and clinical evaluations perhaps every 6–12 weeks for the first 6 months of therapy.

For patients on long-term therapy with efalizumab, 6- to 8-month intervals are optimal for monitoring.

With judicious monitoring, patients on efalizumab can achieve excellent control of their psoriasis for many years.

Alefacept

Mechanism of Action

A fusion protein consisting of the LFA-3 recognition region of CD2 linked to the Fc portion of IgG, alefacept appears to have 1 primary and at least 1 secondary mode of action. CD2 is expressed on all T cells. Attaching to CD2, the exposed Fc portion of alefacept interacts with Fc-γ receptors on natural killer cells resulting in apoptosis [25]. The cells primarily affected are CD45RO+ cells (activator, memory T cells, monocytes, macrophages, and granulocytes), but selectively memory-effector T cells [26, 27]. As CD2 serves a minor costimulatory function during antigen presentation, it is possible that alefacept modifies T cell activation and reactivation [28].

Despite the posited mechanism of action, there appears to be no correlation between response and peripheral CD4 counts [29]. Perhaps the lack of correlation reflects the indiscriminant killing of memory cells instead of effector or memory cells specific to psoriasis.

Studies

The bulk of clinical information on alefacept derives from phase III studies and a single multi-course extension of patients receiving intravenous or intramuscular injections [29–31]. Though the intravenous formulation is no longer available, safety observations in patients treated with intravenous alefacept are pertinent. Alefacept is to be administered weekly for 12 weeks. Hiatus periods of 12 weeks to several months between 12-week courses of therapy are mandated in the product monograph [32].

Monitoring

The only consistent laboratory abnormality found when treating patients with alefacept is suppressed CD4 lymphocyte counts, sometimes profound [33]. According to the product monograph, CD4 counts are taken prior to administration of alefacept and weekly during the 12 weeks of therapy [32]. Should CD4 counts fall below the lower limit of normal, dosing should be withheld until CD4 counts rise. Persistent depression of CD4 counts mandates permanent discontinuation of alefacept.

Product monographs suggest weekly CD4 counts. Personal experience and pragmatic thinking suggests otherwise. Though most patients experience a decline in CD4 counts, few drop below the local laboratory's low-normal limit. It is rare at the approved dose for individuals to experience a precipitous decline in lymphocyte counts. I believe patients and health care resources are better served with CD4 counts done every 2 weeks. As previously noted, low counts require holding of alefacept, while persistently depressed counts necessitate permanent discontinuation.

An overview of data from clinical studies suggests no significant increase in the rate of malignancies or infections in patients treated with alefacept compared to the general population [34]. However, as is the case with recent a meta-analysis, there are too few patients considered over multiple cycles, and adjustments have not been made for drug exposure [31, 35]. A long-term registry program may address these shortcomings (NCT00795353).

Despite some ranking alefacept as the safest of the biological therapies [35], uncertainties remain. We do not know the long-term implications of non-selective depletion of CD2+ cells and memory cells in particular. What happens if at some time in the future, a subject is exposed to or has reactivation of a latent pathogen but has those specific memory cells depleted? Though we know that response and recall of neo-antigen vaccination is intact despite receiving alefacept [23], we do not as yet know the responses in patients receiving more characteristic polyvalent vaccines (NCT00493324).

Summary

Alefacept continues to be used by many patients and prescribed by many clinicians. There appears to be a small subset of psoriasis patients with superlative response [36]. It is unfortunate that a marker for responders remains elusive. For all patients intending to commence treatment with alefacept, a baseline CD4 count is necessary. In accordance with the monograph, weekly CD4 counts are necessary to determine continued dosing. Most patients may administer drug themselves, though the need for careful monitoring of CD4 levels suggests clinic-based administration. Following a 12-week course of therapy, patients may be assessed as needed in order to determine appropriate reintroduction of therapy. The long-term impact of alefacept is not known; consequently, sustained long-term follow-up of patients receiving multiple courses of alefacept or those experiencing persistent depression of CD4 counts is prudent.

References

1 Lebwohl M, Tyring SK, Hamilton TK, Toth D, Glazer S, Tawfik NH, et al: A novel targeted T-cell modulator, efalizumab, for plaque psoriasis. N Engl J Med 2003;349:2004–2013.

2 Leonardi CL: Efalizumab in the treatment of psoriasis. Dermatol Ther 2004;17:393–400.

3 Papp K, Bissonette R, Goldwater R, Ouellet JP, Gratton D, Lynde C, et al: The effective treatment of moderate to severe psoriasis with a new monoclonal antibody. CDA Annu Meet, Vancouver, 1999.

4 Leonardi CL, Papp KA, Gordon KB, Menter A, Feldman SR, Caro I, et al: Extended efalizumab therapy improves chronic plaque psoriasis: results from a randomized phase III trial. J Am Acad Dermatol 2005;52(part 1):425–433.

5 Graves JE, Nunley K, Heffernan MP: Off-label uses of biologics in dermatology: rituximab, omalizumab, infliximab, etanercept, adalimumab, efalizumab, and alefacept (part 2 of 2). J Am Acad Dermatol 2007; 56:e55–e79.

6 Papp KA: Efalizumab: advancing psoriasis management with a novel, targeted T-cell modulator. Drugs Today (Barc) 2004;40:889–899.

7 Davignon D, Martz E, Reynolds T, Kurzinger K, Springer TA: Lymphocyte function-associated antigen 1 (LFA-1): a surface antigen distinct from Lyt-2,3 that participates in T lymphocyte-mediated killing. Proc Natl Acad Sci USA 1981;78:4535–4539.

8 Yang L, Froio RM, Sciuto TE, Dvorak AM, Alon R, Luscinskas FW: ICAM-1 regulates neutrophil adhesion and transcellular migration of TNF-alpha-activated vascular endothelium under flow. Blood 2005;106:584–592.

9 Singer KH, Tuck DT, Sampson HA, Hall RP: Epidermal keratinocytes express the adhesion molecule intercellular adhesion molecule-1 in inflammatory dermatoses. J Invest Dermatol 1989;92: 746–750.

10 Papp KA, Henninger E: Evaluation of efalizumab using safe psoriasis control. BMC Dermatol 2006; 6:8.

11 Papp K, Bissonnette R, Krueger JG, Carey W, Gratton D, Gulliver WP, et al: The treatment of moderate to severe psoriasis with a new anti-CD11a monoclonal antibody. J Am Acad Dermatol 2001; 45:665–674.

12 VHA Pharmacy Benefits Management Strategic Healthcare Group and Medical Advisory Panel: National PBM Drug Monograph: efalizumab (Raptiva). Pharmacy Benefits Management Services, 2004. www.pbm.va.gov/Clinical%20Guidance/Drug%20Monographs/Efalizumab.pdf.

13 Gordon KB, Feldman SR, Koo JY, Menter A, Rolstad T, Krueger G: Definitions of measures of effect duration for psoriasis treatments. Arch Dermatol 2005;141:82–84.

14 European Medicines Agency: Guideline on clinical investigation of medicinal product indicated for the treatment of psoriasis. London, EMEA, 2004. www.emea.europa.eu/pdfs/human/ewp/245402en.pdf.

15 Papp KA, Toth D, Rosoph L: Approaches to discontinuing efalizumab: an open-label study of therapies for managing inflammatory recurrence. BMC Dermatol 2006;6:9.

16 Pincelli C, Henninger E, Casset-Semanaz F: The incidence of arthropathy adverse events in efalizumab-treated patients is low and similar to placebo and does not increase with long-term treatment: pooled analysis of data from phase III clinical trials of efalizumab. Arch Dermatol Res 2006;298:329–338.
17 Papp KA, Shear NH, Poulin Y, Langley RG, Lynde CW: Efficacy and safety of long-term efalizumab therapy: final phase IIIb study results. CDA Annu Meet, Quebec, June 2005.
18 Gottlieb AB, Hamilton T, Caro I, Kwon P, Compton PG, Leonardi CL: Long-term continuous efalizumab therapy in patients with moderate to severe chronic plaque psoriasis: updated results from an ongoing trial. J Am Acad Dermatol 2006;54(suppl 1): S154–S163.
19 Poulin Y, Papp KA, Carey W, Gulliver W, Gupta AK: A favourable benefit/risk ratio with efalizumab: a review of the clinical evidence. J Cutan Med Surg 2006;9(suppl 1):10–17.
20 Gottlieb AB, Gordon KB, Hamilton TK: Maintenance of efficacy and safety with continuous efalizumab therapy in patients with moderate to severe chronic plaque psoriasis: final phase IIIb study results. J Am Acad Dermatol 2005;52(suppl 1): P1.
21 Carey W, Glazer S, Gottlieb AB, Lebwohl M, Leonardi C, Menter A, et al: Relapse, rebound, and psoriasis adverse events: an advisory group report. J Am Acad Dermatol 2006;54(suppl 1):S171–S181.
22 Menter A, Leonardi CL, Sterry W, Bos JD, Papp KA: Long-term management of plaque psoriasis with continuous efalizumab therapy. J Am Acad Dermatol 2006;54(suppl 1):S182–S188.
23 Gottlieb AB, Casale TB, Frankel E, Goffe B, Lowe N, Ochs HD, et al: CD4+ T-cell-directed antibody responses are maintained in patients with psoriasis receiving alefacept: results of a randomized study. J Am Acad Dermatol 2003;49:816–825.
24 Krueger JG, Ochs HD, Patel P, Gilkerson E, Guttman-Yassky E, Dummer W: Effect of therapeutic integrin (CD11a) blockade with efalizumab on immune responses to model antigens in humans: results of a randomized, single blind study. J Invest Dermatol 2008;128:2615–2624.
25 Majeau GR, Meier W, Jimmo B, Kioussis D, Hochman PS: Mechanism of lymphocyte function-associated molecule 3-Ig fusion proteins inhibition of T cell responses: structure/function analysis in vitro and in human CD2 transgenic mice. J Immunol 1994;152:2753–2767.
26 Sanders ME, Makgoba MW, Sharrow SO, Stephany D, Springer TA, Young HA, et al: Human memory T lymphocytes express increased levels of three cell adhesion molecules (LFA-3, CD2, and LFA-1) and three other molecules (UCHL1, CDw29, and Pgp-1) and have enhanced IFN-gamma production. J Immunol 1988;140:1401–1407.
27 da Silva AJ, Brickelmaier M, Majeau GR, Li Z, Su L, Hsu YM, et al: Alefacept, an immunomodulatory recombinant LFA-3/IgG1 fusion protein, induces CD16 signaling and CD2/CD16-dependent apoptosis of CD2(+) cells. J Immunol 2002;168:4462–4471.
28 Miller GT, Hochman PS, Meier W, Tizard R, Bixler SA, Rosa MD, et al: Specific interaction of lymphocyte function-associated antigen 3 with CD2 can inhibit T cell responses. J Exp Med 1993;178:211–222.
29 Krueger GG, Papp KA, Stough DB, Loven KH, Gulliver WP, Ellis CN: A randomized, double-blind, placebo-controlled phase III study evaluating efficacy and tolerability of 2 courses of alefacept in patients with chronic plaque psoriasis. J Am Acad Dermatol 2002;47:821–833.
30 Lebwohl M, Christophers E, Langley R, Ortonne JP, Roberts J, Griffiths CE: An international, randomized, double-blind, placebo-controlled phase 3 trial of intramuscular alefacept in patients with chronic plaque psoriasis. Arch Dermatol 2003;139:719–727.
31 Menter A, Cather JC, Baker D, Farber HF, Lebwohl M, Darif M: The efficacy of multiple courses of alefacept in patients with moderate to severe chronic plaque psoriasis. J Am Acad Dermatol 2006;54: 61–63.
32 VHA Pharmacy Benefits Management Strategic Healthcare Group and Medical Advisory Panel: National PBM Drug Monograph: alefacept. 2003. www.pbm.va.gov/Clinical%20Guidance/Drug%20Monographs/Alefacept.pdf.
33 Ellis CN, Krueger GG: Treatment of chronic plaque psoriasis by selective targeting of memory effector T lymphocytes. N Engl J Med 2001;345:248–255.
34 Jenneck C, Novak N: The safety and efficacy of alefacept in the treatment of chronic plaque psoriasis. Ther Clin Risk Manag 2007;3:411–420.
35 Brimhall AK, King LN, Licciardone JC, Jacobe H, Menter A: Safety and efficacy of alefacept, efalizumab, etanercept and infliximab in treating moderate to severe plaque psoriasis: a meta-analysis of randomized controlled trials. Br J Dermatol 2008; 159:274–285.
36 Canadian Agency for Drugs and Technologies in Health: CEDAC final recommendations on reconsideration and reasons for recommendation: alefacept resubmission. 2006. www.cadth.ca/media/cdr/complete/cdr_complete_Amevive_Resubmission_Sept-27-06.pdf.

Addendum and Cautionary Note

There are many learning points, but an important conclusion can be made with respect the withdrawal of efalizumab from the European and Canadian markets in February [1, 2] and from the USA and other markets in April 2009 [3]: the warning systems work. The adverse-event reporting systems established by the major medicinal regulatory agencies, and coordinated by the International Conference on Harmonization [4], functioned effectively and appropriately in this case. Safety and risk are relative; they are dependent on vigilant observation, dispassionate analysis, and context. Here, I will reconstruct an approximate risk-benefit analysis and outline an approach for future models.

There have been a total of 7 phase I studies conducted on efalizumab [5], including the 1998 first-in-man study involving 31 participants each receiving a single infusion of efalizumab ranging from 0.03 to 10.0 mg/kg [6]. With the additional 2 phase II studies and 7 phase III studies, 3,291 subjects had been exposed to efalizumab in clinical trials by 2004 [5]. The incidence of malignancies, infections, and serious infections was comparable between efalizumab and placebo [5, 6]. Withdrawal was based upon 3 confirmed cases of progressive multifocal leukoencephalopathy (PML) [7]: 2 cases aged 70 years or older and using efalizumab for more than 4 years (reported in September 2008 and October 2008, respectively), both died; 1 case aged 47 years and using efalizumab for more than 3 years (reported January 2009), outcome unknown. At the time of withdrawal, approximately 46,000 patients had been exposed to efalizumab. Of these, 14,000 had been exposed for longer than 1 year, 5,100 for longer than 2 years, and 1,900 for longer than 3 years [8].

The foregoing data can be used to generate a study on the statistical analysis of risk. Estimates of the rate of events, PML in this instance, from the Poisson distribution (an exact calculation) and the frequency of events using the binomial distribution (approximate) [9] are presented in table 1. A total of 31 subjects were treated in the first phase I study conducted in 1998. By 2004, more than 3,000 patients had received at least 1 dose of efalizumab. The low limits of the CI for rates and frequencies are acceptable, until there is an event. Much like any activity, everything is perfectly safe until something happens. Once an event occurs, it is necessary to determine what the background rate is for that event. Though we do not know the incidence of PML in a normal population, we expect it to be rare, less than 0.0001. In 2008, prior to the first 2 PML cases , an argument could be made that the overall risk of PML was low, except in patients on efalizumab for more than 3 years; those particularly at risk were the elderly patients on efalizumab for more than 3 years. Note the significant increase in rate CI for 0, 2 and 3 PML cases: 0–3.68, 0.24–7.23, and 0.619–8.77, with corresponding frequency CI for patients on treatment for 3 or more years: 0–0.002, 0.0003–0.004, and 0.0006–0.005, respectively. The third case implies the incidence of PML in patients treated with efalizumab for 3 years or more is at least 6-fold higher that expected.

The cautionary note is a 'Catch-22'. Safety is a relative value. Longer and greater experience implies more confidence. More confidence implies a safer product. Delays stifle advancement, innovation, and societal benefit [10]. Poorly considered regulations produce conflicting outcomes, increased cost, and suboptimal utility [10, 11]. PML was an unexpected, unfortunate, and unforeseen event associated with the treatment of efalizumab. The association between PML and efalizumab is undeniable. Despite the benefit brought to thousands of patients, efalizumab was seen to provide too great a risk for the benefit provided. Efalizumab was a safe and effective drug; it just was not safe enough.

A better model for safety data is to provide CI for events occurring in the treated and comparator populations. Significant overlap informs us that differences are not likely to be significant. When the upper boundaries of 1 population are close to the lower bounds of another, we are more inclined to consider the differences noteworthy. Even in cases where a comparator is not available, CI provide some guidance on the likelihood of an unwanted event. Safety is all about confidence.

Table 1. CI for PML rates (Poisson) and frequencies (binomial) of PML in total and selected populations of efalizumab-treated patients at development and post-marketing epochs

	Population in blocks of time				Population according to drug exposure		
	drug exposure	n	Poisson CI	binomial CI	drug exposure	n	binomial CI
1998		31	0–3.7	0–0.1			
2004		03,291	0–3.68	0–0.001			
2008[1]	total n	46,000	0–3.6889	0–0.0001	<1 year	32,000	0–0.0001
	>1 year	14,000	0–3.689	0–0.0003	1–2 years	08,900	0–0.0004
	>2 years	05,100	0–3.68	0–0.0007	2–3 years	03,200	0–0.0012
	>3 years	01,900	0–3.68	0–0.0019			
2008[2]	total n	46,000	0.2422–7.2247	0.0000–0.0002	<1 year	32,000	0.0000–0.0002
(2 PML cases)	>1 year	14,000	0.242–7.225	0.0000–0.0005	1–2 years	08,900	0.0001–0.0008
	>2 years	05,100	0.242–7.225	0.0001–0.0014	2–3 years	03,200	0.0002–0.0023
	>3 years	1,900	0.242–7.225	0.0003–0.0038			
	< 1						
	1–2						
2009[3]	total n	46,000	0.6187–8.7673	0.0000–0.0002	<1 year	32,000	0.0000–0.0003
(3 PML cases)	>1 year	14,000	0.6189–8.767	0.0001–0.0006	1–2 years	08,900	0.0001–0.0010
	>2 years	05,100	0.6189–8.767	0.0002–0.0017	2–3 years	03,200	0.0003–0.0027
	>3 years	01,900	0.6189–8.767	0.0006–0.0046			

[1] Period immediately prior to the first 2 reported cases of PML.
[2] Period following the first 2 reports.
[3] Period following the third confirmed case.

References

1 European Medicines Agency: Questions and answers on the recommendation to suspend the marketing authorisation for Raptiva (EMEA/CHMP/15525/ 2009). London, EMEA, 2009. www.emea.europa.eu/humandocs/PDFs/EPAR/raptiva/RaptivaQ&A_ 1552509en.pdf (accessed May 8, 2009).

2 Health Canada: Suspension of marketing of Raptiva (efalizumab) in Canada. www.hc-sc.gc.ca/dhp-mps/medeff/advisories-avis/prof/_2009/raptiva_2_hpc-cps-eng.php. Ottawa, Health Canada, 2009 (accessed May 8, 2009).

3 Genetech: Genentech announces voluntary withdrawal of Raptiva from the US Market. San Francisco, Genetech, 2009. www.gene.com/gene/products/information/immunological/raptiva (accessed May 8, 2009).

4 International Conference on Harmonisation of Technical Requirements for Registration of Pharmaceuticals for Human Use: Post-approval safety data management: definitions and standards for expedited reporting E2D. Geneve, ICH, 2003. www.ich.org/LOB/media/MEDIA631.pdf (accessed May 8, 2009).

5 European Medicines Agency: Scientific discussion (Raptiva). London, EMEA, 2004. www.emea.europa.eu/humandocs/PDFs/EPAR/raptiva/6565604en6.pdf (accessed May 8, 2009).

6 Food and Drug Administration: Biological license application STN BL 125075/0 for efalizumab for the treatment of moderate to severe chronic plaque psoriasis. Silver Spring, FDA, 2003. www.fda.gov/ohrms/dockets/ac/03/briefing/3983B1_02_FDA-Raptiva.pdf (accessed May 8, 2009).

7 Reuters: EMD Serono Canada Inc.: Health Canada Recommends Suspension of Raptiva(R) in Canada. Retuers, 2009. www.reuters.com/article/pressRelease/idUS198878+23-Feb-2009+MW20090223 (accessed May 8, 2009)
8 Genetech: Raptiva prescribing information. San Francisco, Genetech, 2009. www.gene.com/gene/products/information/pdf/raptiva-prescribing.pdf (accessed May 8, 2009).
9 Fleiss JL, Levin B, Paik MC: Statistical Methods for Rates and Proportions. Hoboken, John Wiley and Sons, 2003.
10 Tewksbury JG, Crandall MS, Crane WE: Measuring the societal benefits of innovation. Science 1980;209:658-662.
11 Lave LB: Conflicting objective in regulating the automobile. Science 1981;212:893-899.

K.A. Papp, MD
Probity Medical Research
135 Union Street East
Waterloo, ON N2J 1C4 (Canada)
Tel. +1 519 579 9535, Fax +1 519 679 8312, E-Mail kapapp@probitymedical.com

Yawalkar N (ed): Management of Psoriasis.
Curr Probl Dermatol. Basel, Karger, 2009, vol 38, pp 107–136

Management of Severe Psoriasis with TNF Antagonists

Adalimumab, Etanercept and Infliximab

Rotraut Mössner[a] · Kristian Reich[b]

[a]Department of Dermatology, Georg August University, Göttingen, and [b]Dermatologikum Hamburg, Hamburg, Germany

Abstract

Three specific tumor necrosis factor (TNF) antagonists, adalimumab, etanercept and infliximab, have been approved for the treatment of psoriasis. Their efficacy, not only in psoriasis but also in psoriatic arthritis, has been demonstrated in large prospective randomized placebo-controlled trials. At present, the discussion about the use of these drugs is dominated by issues of the risk-benefit ratio and by economic considerations. In this chapter, we give an introduction to the different TNF antagonists, with the main focus on therapy management and safety issues.

Tumor necrosis factor-α (TNF-α) play a central role in the pathophysiology of a variety of chronic inflammatory diseases, including psoriasis, psoriatic arthritis, inflammatory bowel disease, ankylosing spondylitis and rheumatoid arthritis. This role of TNF-α has been underscored recently by the therapeutic success of therapies specifically targeting this cytokine. So far, three TNF antagonists, adalimumab, etanercept and infliximab, have been licensed in the therapy of plaque-type psoriasis. In the European Union, they are indicated in plaque psoriasis for 'second-line' use, i.e. only for patients in whom other systemic therapies were ineffective, had to be discontinued due to side effects or were contraindicated. In contrast, in the USA, infliximab has a 'conditional' first-line approval, and may be used in patients with chronic severe (i.e. extensive and/or disabling) plaque psoriasis who are candidates for systemic therapy and when other systemic therapies are medically less appropriate. Etanercept has a first-line approval in the USA in patients with chronic moderate-to-severe plaque psoriasis, who are candidates for systemic therapies or phototherapy.

The efficacy of the TNF antagonists has been demonstrated in numerous randomized placebo-controlled double-blind trials. The discussion on therapy with

TNF antagonists is currently dominated by issues of risk-benefit, cost effectiveness and patient selection (e.g. first-line vs. second-line indication of TNF antagonists). Furthermore, experience in distinct patient subgroups, for example in patients with significant comorbidities such as renal insufficiency, is increasing, and these new treatments may become available to patient subgroups that only have very limited treatment options at the moment. In this chapter, we want to give an overview of the TNF antagonists licensed in the therapy of plaque-type psoriasis, about safety issues and therapy management.

Structures and Properties of TNF Antagonists

All of the TNF antagonists bind their well-defined target molecules with high affinity and specificity, and interfere with the pathomechanism of inflammatory diseases characterized by TNF overproduction on the basis of inhibitory, neutralizing and/or cytotoxic activity. Relevant properties of TNF antagonists are described here, and are summarized in table 1.

Structures

Infliximab is a chimeric monoclonal antibody. The variable regions are of murine origin and are coupled to human IgG1 κ constant domains. Adalimumab is a fully human IgG1 monoclonal antibody. Like infliximab, adalimumab neutralizes the biologic activities of TNF by blocking its interactions with the p55 and p75 cell surface receptors; thus, modulating TNF-dependent biologic responses. Etanercept is a human fusion protein consisting of 2 molecules of the extracellular domains of the p75 TNF receptor and the constant fragment of IgG1.

Pharmacodynamics

TNF-α is active as a homotrimer, but it is also bound as monomer, dimer or trimer to the surface of TNF-α-producing cells. Infliximab binds to all forms of soluble and membrane-bound TNF-α with high specificity, but unlike the TNF-antagonistic fusion protein etanercept, it does not bind lymphotoxin-α (TNF-β; table 1). The concept that infliximab is also able to at least partially antagonize receptor-bound TNF-α is based on the high affinity of infliximab to TNF-α, and on the documented high association-dissociation rate of TNF-α at the TNF receptor. Both infliximab and TNF are multivalent proteins: in a situation of antigen excess, 1 infliximab molecule can bind 2 different TNF trimers, while, in antibody excess, 3 infliximab molecules can bind to 1 TNF trimer. The high affinity due to the formation of large immune complexes,

Table 1. Important characteristics of TNF antagonists used in the treatment of psoriasis

	Infliximab (Remicade®) [5, 16, 17, 57, 58, 61, 62]	Etanercept (Enbrel®) [39, 59, 60, 63, 105–107]	Adalimumab (Humira®) [10, 22, 37, 38, 59, 64]
Molecule	• Chimeric IgG1/κ monoclonal antibody	• p75-IgG1 Fc-fragment fusion protein	• Human IgG1/κ monoclonal antibody
Target structure	• TNF-α	• TNF-α • Lymphotoxin-α (TNF-β)	• TNF-α
Regulatory affairs	• Moderate-to-severe plaque psoriasis • Psoriatic arthritis (in combination with methotrexate, if possible)	• Moderate-to-severe plaque psoriasis (approved for 24 weeks only) • Psoriatic arthritis	• Moderate-to-severe plaque psoriasis • Psoriatic arthritis
Dose/route of administration	• 5 mg/kg body weight as i.v. infusion, weeks 0, 2 and 6, then every 8 weeks	• 2 × 25 mg/week or 1 × 50 mg s.c. • 2 × 50 mg/week allowed during the first 12 weeks in plaque psoriasis	• 80 mg s.c. week 0, 40 mg s.c. week 1, then 40 mg s.c. every other week in plaque psoriasis; • 40 mg s.c. every other week in psoriatic arthritis
Pharmacokinetics	• Bioavailability (i.v.): 100% • C_{max} (5 mg/kg): 118 μg/ml • Half-life (single dose): 8–9.5 days • Half-life (steady state): several weeks	• Bioavailability (s.c.): 76% • C_{max} (25 mg): 1.7 ± 0.7 μg/ml • Half-life (single dose): ~70 h • Half-life (steady state): ~100 h	• Bioavailability (s.c.): 64% • C_{max} (40 mg): 4.7 ± 1.6 μg/ml • Half-life (single dose): 14 days
Efficacy in psoriasis	• PASI 75: week 10: ~76–88%, week 24: ~80%	• PASI 75: • 2 × 25 mg/week: week 12: ~35% week 24: ~50% • 1 × 50 mg/week: week 12: 37% week 24: 71% • 2 × 50 mg/week: week 12: ~50% week 24: ~60%	• PASI 75: • Loading dose week 0: 80 mg, then 40 mg every other week week 16: 71–80% week 24: ~70%
Long-term efficacy	• PASI 75: week 50: ~60%	• PASI 75: 2 × 50mg/week[a] week 60: ~60%	• PASI 75 week 60: ~56%
Efficacy in psoriatic arthritis	• Good efficacy; long-term treatment reduces progress of bone destruction • ACR 20 response: weeks 14–16: ~60% week 24: 54% week 50: 69%	• Good efficacy; long-term treatment reduces progress of bone destruction • ACR 20 response week 12: 59%, week 24: ~60%, weeks ~48–60: ~64%	• Good efficacy; long-term treatment reduces progress of bone destruction ACR 20 response week 12: 58%, week 24: 57% week 48: 56%

[a] This dose is only approved for the first 12 weeks of treatment, after week 12 only the doses 1 × 50 or 2 × 25 mg/week are approved.

referred to as avidity, significantly reduces the possibility that bioactive TNF can dissociate from infliximab. The ability of infliximab to bind to membrane-bound TNF-α in this fashion appears to be linked to additional effects on TNF-α-producing cells (apoptosis, complement lysis, antibody-dependent cellular cytotoxicity), which have been described in vitro [1] and in vivo [2] and have been proposed to contribute to the clinical efficacy of infliximab [3].

Binding properties of adalimumab are similar to those of infliximab. Each adalimumab molecule can bind up to 2 TNF trimers, and a single TNF trimer can bind up to 3 molecules of adalimumab. Adalimumab does not bind lymphotoxin-α (TNF-β). Less is known about the ability of adalimumab to induce cell-depleting effects, but, based on structural similarities to infliximab, it is conceivable that adalimumab may induce apoptosis, complement lysis and antibody-dependent cellular cytotoxicity.

Unlike infliximab and adalimumab, etanercept binds not only to TNF-α, but also to lymphotoxin-α (TNF-β). It is believed that the bivalent etanercept binds trimeric TNF at a ratio of 1:1, with the consequence that 1 binding site for the TNF receptor remains unoccupied. In vitro analyses indicate a reduced stability of etanercept-TNF complexes compared to infliximab-TNF complexes, as well as remaining biologic activity of TNF released from the etanercept-TNF complexes. Etanercept is believed to bind only soluble and membrane-bound TNF trimers, but not monomers and dimers. Even though etanercept contains the Fc portion of IgG1, it does not appear to fix complement. It is also speculated that, due to the different binding properties of etanercept compared to infliximab, the former is unlikely to form aggregates on the surface of TNF-producing cells that can activate complement-dependent lysis and antibody-dependent cell-mediated cytotoxicity.[4] The clinical effect of the binding of etanercept to lymphotoxin-α is not clear.

Pharmacokinetics and Metabolism

Infliximab is administered as a short intravenous infusion over a period of at least 2 h at a total dose of 5 mg/kg body weight. According to the label for plaque psoriasis, infusions are given at weeks 0, 2 and 6 at the beginning, and then every 8 weeks for maintenance therapy (table 1). In psoriasis, infliximab is indicated for monotherapy, while in rheumatologic conditions (including psoriatic arthritis) infliximab is often used in combination with methotrexate, a regimen that has not been investigated systematically in psoriasis yet. The mean elimination half-life is ~8.5–9 days; however, depending on the dose and the duration of treatment, infliximab can be detected in the serum for up to 28 weeks.

It appears that the ability to build up a stable preinfusion (steady-state) serum concentration of infliximab during regular long-term treatment is associated with the maintenance of clinical response in most patients [5]. The factors responsible for interindividual differences in the long-term pharmacokinetics of infliximab and other biologics are presently not fully understood, but the presence of antidrug antibodies has been shown to be associated with an accelerated infliximab clearance [6].

There is evidence that the pharmacokinetic characteristics of infliximab are typical of intravenous immunoglobulin G_1 [6]. It is generally believed that catabolism of IgG antibodies directed against soluble antigens is mediated by the reticulo-endothelial system and is independent of enzymatic systems frequently involved in drug metabolism, such as the cytochrom P450 isozymes [7].

Adalimumab has been approved in the indication of plaque psoriasis at a dose of 80 mg s.c. week 0, 40 mg week 1 and 40 mg every other week thereafter. Interestingly, mean steady-state trough concentrations vary between patients without and with concomitant methotrexate (approximately 5 and 8 to 9 µg/ml, respectively), and methotrexate reduced adalimumab apparent clearance after single and multiple dosing by 29 and 44%, respectively [8].

The mean half-life of adalimumab was approximately 2 weeks, ranging from 10 to 20 days [4, 9]. No pharmacokinetic data are available in patients with renal or hepatic impairment. As in the case of infliximab, population pharmacokinetic analysis indicates a trend toward a higher apparent clearance of adalimumab in the presence of anti-adalimumab antibodies.

Etanercept is applied in the therapy of plaque psoriasis at a dose of 25 mg s.c. twice weekly or 50 mg s.c. once weekly. For the first 12 weeks of treatment, the dose may be doubled to 50 mg twice weekly. Treatment with etanercept in plaque psoriasis has been approved for 24 weeks only. The half-life of etanercept is about 70 h. As opposed to adalimumab, etanercept clearance was not affected by concurrent administration of methotrexate. Little is known about the metabolism of etanercept, but it seems to be unaffected by renal function and no unchanged drug is found in the urine.

Clinical Efficacy of TNF Antagonists

The clinical efficacy of the 3 TNF antagonists has been demonstrated in large prospective randomized placebo-controlled trials (table 1). While all 3 drugs have proved efficacious, however, there are some differences between the drugs. The response rate, as measured in percent of patients obtaining at least a 75% reduction in the Psoriasis Area and Severity Index (PASI) compared to baseline (PASI 75) at the end of the induction phase (approx. weeks 10–16), was higher in infliximab- and adalimumab-treated patients compared to patients treated with etanercept. This corresponds to a shorter time needed to achieve a mean reduction in PASI of 50% in infliximab and adalimumab-treated patients, a response regarded as clinically relevant. In the infliximab and adalimumab studies, a mean reduction in the PASI of 50% was observed within approximately 2–5 weeks, compared to about 6–12 weeks in etanercept-treated patients, depending on the dose used.

However, in the course of a longer treatment period of about 6 months, PASI 75 values differ less between the TNF antagonists as values decrease to 70–80% in patients treated with adalimumab and infliximab, and increase to 50%–70% in patients treated with etanercept. During a treatment period of 1 year, PASI 75 values were ~60% in infliximab and adalimumab-treated patients, while no trials evaluating PASI after 1 year of therapy are available for etanercept. For a clinical example of the efficacy of a TNF-antagonist therapy, see figure 1.

Head-to-Head Trials of TNF Antagonists

So far, in plaque psoriasis, a single head-to-head trial of a TNF antagonist with classical therapies has been conducted. Adalimumab was tested against methotrexate and placebo in a controlled randomized double-blind trial with a duration of 16 weeks, including 271 patients who were naive both to treatment with TNF antagonists and methotrexate [10]. Adalimumab was used in the approved dosing scheme, and for methotrexate a dose escalation scheme was applied starting from 7.5 mg/week, in which a maximum dose of 25 mg/week could be reached from week 12 onwards. Patients who achieved a PASI 50 response at week 8 or 12 were not eligible for further dose escalation and were treated with a maximum dose of 15 or 20 mg/week, respectively. After 16 weeks, adalimumab treatment was superior to methotrexate and placebo, with 79.6% of patients treated with adalimumab, compared to 35.5% of patients treated with methotrexate and 18.9% of placebo-treated patients achieving a PASI 75 response. As in other clinical trials with methotrexate, a protocol using a dose-escalation scheme probably did not allow sufficient time for all potential therapy responders to be identified, as the higher doses of 20 mg or 25 mg/week were usually reached only after week 8, but it is unlikely that a longer treatment period would have had a major impact on the results. So far, no trials comparing different TNF antagonists have been conducted.

Effects on Quality of Life

The effects of TNF antagonists on quality of life have been investigated in several studies. The Dermatology Life Quality Index is frequently employed in clinical trials as a measure of disease-specific quality of life. Generally, patients treated with TNF antagonists showed a significant improvement in disease-associated quality of life as compared to the placebo-treated groups [11]. In a meta-analysis of adalimumab treatment in plaque-psoriasis, it could also be shown that the improvement in the Dermatology Life Quality Index was significantly higher in the subgroup achieving at least a PASI 90 response compared to those patients with a PASI 75 response only [12]. This indicates that even patients who respond well to therapy but are not almost/completely free of disease retain a certain impairment in disease-related quality of life.

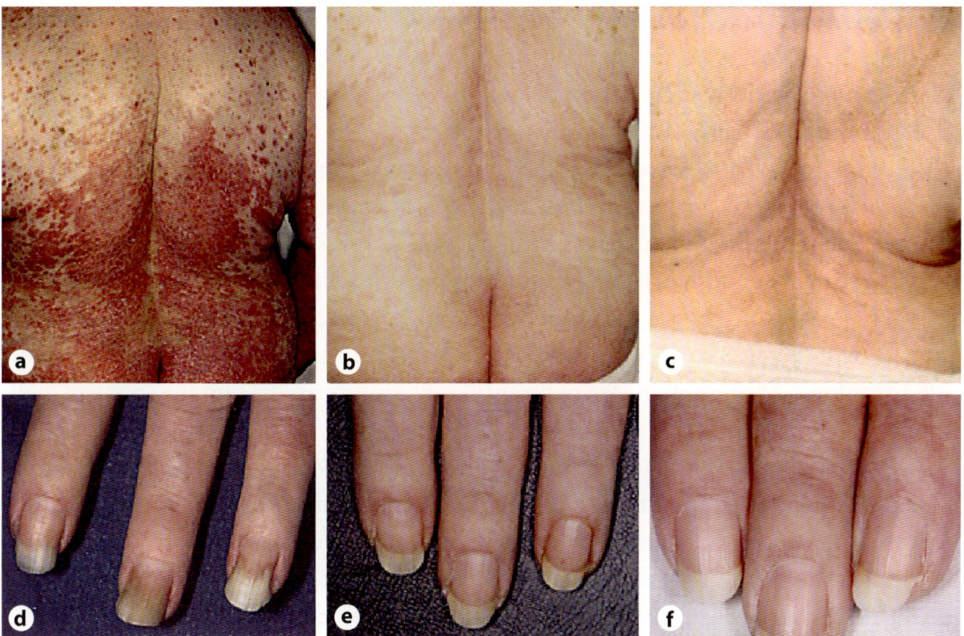

Fig. 1. Improvement in psoriatic skin and nail disease under infliximab therapy at 5 mg/kg body weight according to the standard dosing scheme, shown before therapy (**a**, **d**) and after week 4 (**b**), week 24 (**d**) and 1 year of therapy (**c**, **f**).

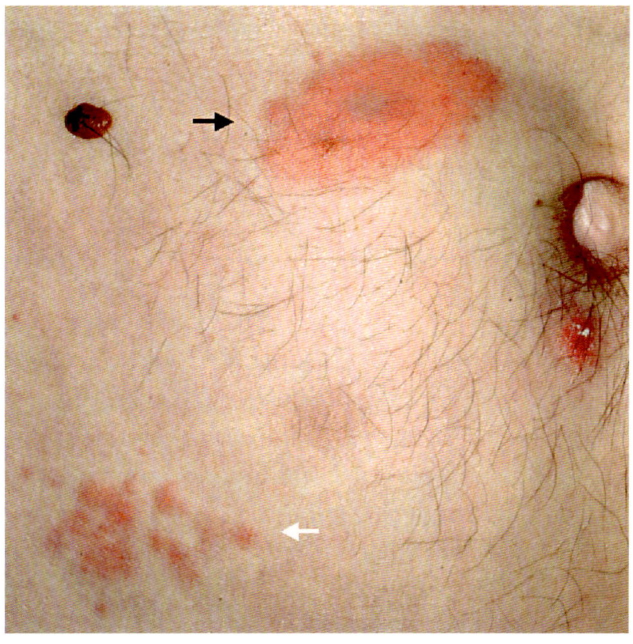

Fig. 2. Injection reaction (black arrow) manifesting 3 days after the fourth injection of etanercept 50 mg s.c. as edematous erythematous plaque around the injection site on the abdomen of a 38-year-old male psoriasis patient in the second week of treatment. At the injection site of the preceding injection (white arrow), partially confluent red papules developed concomitantly. Over the following 3 months, reaction at the injection sites decreased in intensity and finally ceased completely.

Safety and Tolerability

There is a continuously increasing amount of safety data available for TNF antagonists based on the use of TNF antagonists in psoriasis and in their other indications, such as rheumatoid arthritis, ankylosing spondylitis and inflammatory bowel disease.

The overall safety profile of TNF antagonists seems similar in all indications. However, it can not currently be excluded that certain safety aspects, such as the risk of skin cancer and hepatopathy, differ in patients with plaque-type psoriasis due to previous exposure to UV phototherapy, and also because of differences in these patients with regard to comorbidities and prior immunosuppressive therapies or comedications. At present, there are no sufficient long-term data on the safety of TNF antagonists in patients with plaque psoriasis.

Key safety considerations of TNF antagonists include common side effects, mainly infections including rare but important opportunistic infections, in particular tuberculosis, and infusion/injection reactions. The relationship between TNF antagonists and some other significant events that have been infrequently observed during treatment, including cases of severe liver toxicity, demyelinating diseases or lymphoma, is less clear and therefore caution is recommended. Most data on TNF-antagonist-associated risks stem from comparisons of TNF-antagonist-treated patients with patients receiving disease-modifying antirheumatic drugs (DMARD) with or without glucocorticosteroids in rheumatologic indications and in inflammatory bowel disease. In an analysis of large Spanish registries of patients suffering from rheumatoid arthritis, and of a US registry on patients with Crohn's disease (TREAT), mortality was not increased in patients treated with TNF antagonists compared to patients not receiving anti-TNF treatment [13].

The overall pattern of safety issues appears to be similar among TNF-α-antagonists that are used for the treatment of psoriasis and psoriatic arthritis patients, except for infusion/injection reactions and, possibly, the frequency of certain opportunistic infections, such as tuberculosis.

Infusion and Injection Reactions

Acute reactions during or within 24 h after infusion of infliximab are distinguished from delayed reactions occurring between 24 h and 14 days after the infusion [14]. Classification of mild, moderate and severe reactions is usually applied to acute infusion reactions [15]. Acute infusion reactions (defined in clinical trials as any reaction during or within 1–2 h after the infusion) were the most frequent reasons for discontinuation of therapy in clinical trials (2.8% discontinuation rate in all clinical trials). Infusion reactions were observed in about 3–7% of infusions with infliximab compared to 1–2% of infusions with placebo [16, 17]. The majority of infusion reactions were mild to moderate, with symptoms such as flush, pruritus, chill, headache and urticaria, while severe infusion reactions were rare (<0.3%). Severe acute infusion reactions with airway involvement (bronchial spasm) and/or marked cardiovascular reactions occurred in about 1% of the patients treated in clinical trials with infliximab (placebo: 0%) and in 0.1% of the infusions with infliximab [18]. The underlying mechanisms of acute infusion reactions – IgE-mediated anaphylactic reactions or non-IgE-mediated reactions – are not entirely clear. Increased IgE titers or serum tryptase levels were not detected in patients treated with infliximab for Crohn's disease who experienced acute infusion reactions (n = 11) [19]. In most cases, re-treatment with infliximab was possible after preventive treatment, a fact also arguing against an IgE-mediated mechanism [19]. In case of mild or moderate acute infusion reaction, it is recommended to interrupt the infusion, infuse physiologic saline, treat with antihistamines and paracetamol/acetaminophen, and then restart the infliximab infusion at an initially reduced rate. After severe infusion reactions, infliximab therapy should be discontinued. A detailed recommendation for a severity-adapted procedure can be found in Cheifetz and Mayer [15]. In patients with prior infusion reactions, pretreatment with oral antihistamines, paracetamol/acetaminophen and/or glucocorticosteroids should also be considered for future infusions. Approximately 5% of infusion reactions are confined to the administration site, include swelling or pain, and are usually mild.

Acute infusion reactions seem to be more frequent in patients with antibodies directed against infliximab (ATI; antibodies against the murine part of the protein, present in up to 28% of psoriatic patients receiving infliximab monotherapy) than in patients in whom such antibodies were not detected [18, 20]. Routine determination of infliximab-directed antibodies cannot be performed presently. Accumulating evidence suggests that particularly patients receiving infliximab irregularly or with prolonged treatment-free intervals without additional immunosuppressive therapy (such as methotrexate) are at increased risk of developing ATI and, possibly, associated infusion reactions [17]. In rare cases, delayed infusion reactions [serum-sickness-like (type III) reactions characterized by generalized exanthema, myalgia, diffuse arthralgia and fever, and presumably induced by soluble circulating immune complexes] may occur after infliximab treatment. Delayed infusion reactions were observed more frequently in patients who had interrupted infliximab therapy for a prolonged period of time, and an association with ATI development is probable. Thus, the frequency is about 0.2% of patients receiving regular therapy, while retrospective analyses indicated increased rates dependent on the length of therapy-free intervals (e.g. 5.3% of patients with an infusion interval between 2 and 11 months). Continuation of therapy with infliximab in patients with a delayed infusion reaction is not recommended.

Injection Reactions in Therapy with Etanercept and Adalimumab

Acute hypersensitivity reactions under therapy with etanercept or adalimumab are rare (<1/100), while injection reactions on the site of application are observed more frequently [14]. In clinical trials, they were more frequent in psoriatic patients treated with etanercept (14%) as compared to placebo-treated patients (6%). They typically manifest as itching and erythema around the injection site, sometimes accompanied by edematous swelling or papules (fig. 2). The injection site reactions manifest within the first weeks of treatment, in most cases 1 or 2 days after injection, and persist for 3–5 days. The intensity of the reactions tends to decline with continuing injections. The injection site reactions are thought to constitute T-cell-mediated delayed-type hypersensitivity reactions with consecutive tolerance induction. The cellular dermal infiltrate is dominated by $CD8^+$ cytotoxic T cells [21]. In older injections sites, the injection reactions may reoccur, which has been interpreted as a recall phenomenon. Therapy with etanercept can usually be continued when typical injection site reactions occur, and topical therapy with mid-potent corticosteroids for several days can be initiated starting immediately after the injection.

Injection site reactions to adalimumab occurred in 6.6% of patients receiving adalimumab and in 3.1% of placebo-treated psoriatic arthritis patients in a clinical trial in which 50% of the patients were concomitantly treated with methotrexate [22]. In a phase II trial with adalimumab in patients with plaque psoriasis, injection reactions occurred in less than 5% of patients in a treatment interval of 60 weeks and no patient discontinued the study drug as a consequence of injection reactions [23]. Antibodies directed against adalimumab have not been reported to be associated with an increased rate of adverse events.

Infections

Infections are the most common adverse events reported in spontaneous post-launch reports of TNF antagonists. There seems to be an increased risk associated with TNF-antagonist treatment for (serious) skin and soft tissue infections, for bacterial intracellular infections and for granulomatous infections.

Results from several European registries suggest an increased risk of infections in patients treated with TNF inhibitors, with a decreasing trend with ongoing therapy explained by an increase in the first months of therapy [24]. Based on published reports of clinical trials, there has been no consistent estimation of the overall risk for serious infection associated with anti-TNF therapy. A meta-analysis of placebo-controlled clinical trials with infliximab and adalimumab estimated the odds ratio for serious infections of the TNF-antagonist-treated groups to be 2.0 (95% CI: 1.3–3.1) [25]. There are, however, some limitations of this analysis, such as the fact that TNF antagonist dosages used in several of the treatment groups were higher than those approved at present. In contrast, data from a large prospective registry including 7,664 anti-TNF-treated patients and 1,354 DMARD-treated patients with severe rheumatoid arthritis from Great Britain yielded an incidence rate ratio (adjusted for baseline risk) that was similar among the patient groups. However, the risk for serious skin and soft tissue infections was increased in the anti-TNF-treated patients, with an adjusted incidence rate ratio of 4.28 (95% CI: 1.06–17.17), and serious bacterial intracellular infections (n = 19), mostly with *Mycobacterium tuberculosis*, *Legionella pneumophila* and *Salmonella species*, occurred exclusively in TNF-antagonist-treated patients [26]. Data from a recent retrospective survey conducted in France provide further evidence for a higher risk of *Legionella pneumophila* pneumonia in patients receiving TNF antagonists compared to the general population [27].

Other granulomatous infections that have been reported in association with TNF antagonists include infections due to *Histoplasma capsulatum*, *Cryptococcus neoformans*, *Coccidioides inmitis*, *Aspergillus* and *Listeria monocytogenes* [reviewed in 4].

Granuloma formation is a typical defense mechanism against intracellular pathogens that is orchestrated by TNF-α, and its inhibition is likely to contribute to the increased tuberculosis risk seen with infliximab, adalimumab, and – probably to a lower extent – with etanercept [28]. Tuberculosis is the most frequent granulomatous infection occurring under anti-TNF treatment. The time-to-onset of tuberculosis was considerably shorter in patients treated with infliximab compared to those receiving etanercept according to data from a voluntary reporting system established by the Food and Drug Administration (FDA), the Adverse Events Reporting System. While 43% of cases of tuberculosis associated with infliximab occurred within the first 90 days of treatment, in patients treated with etanercept, tuberculosis occurred more uniformly during the evaluated reporting period, with only 10% of cases occurring during the first 90 days of treatment [29]. The majority of patients treated with anti-TNF agents who developed active tuberculosis experienced extrapulmonary manifestations, and almost 25% had disseminated disease [reviewed in 30]. The evaluation of data from Spanish registries (starting April 2002) demonstrated the benefit of a consequent adherence to tuberculosis screening and treatment recommendations [31]. Only 2 patients developed active tuberculosis within the group of patients in whom guidelines were strictly followed (4,546 patient-years), compared to 13 patients where this was not the case (4,170 patient-years). Interestingly, when considering only the patient population treated with TNF antagonists in whom the first Mendel-Mantoux test was positive (≥5 mm), only 1 out of 950 patients who received isoniacide treatment developed active tuberculosis compared to 1 out of 50 patients in whom no isoniacide was given. In 6 patients who had developed active tuberculosis under therapy with TNF antagonists in France, TNF antagonists were re-initiated after completion of anti-tuberculosis therapy, and none of these patients suffered a relapse of active tuberculosis within the mean follow-up time of 42.7 months (range 18–60 months) [32]. This suggests that in such patients with a very high need for therapy, re-initiation of TNF antagonists may be considered after consequent antituberculosis therapy.

Potential recipients of TNF antagonists should be rigorously screened for tuberculosis with a detailed medical history, questioning about potential tuberculosis exposure (including recent travel and skin testing), assessment for symptoms (such as cough and weight loss) and a chest radiography. Patient surveillance and monitoring during treatment should take into account the fact that symptoms such as fever and an increase in acute phase proteins as serologic indicators can be suppressed during anti-TNF therapy. Particular care should be taken when patients come from areas where certain opportunistic infections are endemic. As with other immunosuppressive drugs, TNF antagonists should not be given to patients with active infections.

Antinuclear Antibodies and Lupus-Erythematosus-Like Symptoms

Antinuclear antibodies (ANA) may appear de novo under therapy with TNF antagonists. The titer of these ANA is frequently low (e.g. 1:40) and may vary or fall below detection levels. Manifestation of higher titers of ANA (e.g. ≥1:320) and of anti-dsDNA antibodies is observed less frequently, and factors such as different underlying diseases or methods of detection complicate the comparison of values between studies. Only a small subgroup of patients who develop autoantibodies develop lupus erythematosus (LE)-like symptoms [33, 34]. Autoantibodies usually disappear within months after termination of the anti-TNF therapy [34]. A routine determination of ANA under therapy with TNF antagonists is not necessary. Therapy with TNF antagonists may be continued in the presence of ANA when no associated clinical symptoms are present.

A retrospective analysis has estimated the proportion of patients who develop LE-like symptoms under therapy with the TNF antagonists to amount to about 0.2% for both infliximab and etanercept [35]. In this study, in about half of the patients symptoms were limited to the skin (n = 10), and comprised a heterogeneous spectrum of symptoms including purpura, exanthema, increased photosensitivity, chilblain lesions and butterfly erythema. The symptoms resolved in all cases within 1 month after discontinuation of anti-TNF therapy [35]. The other half of the affected patients (n = 12) presented with symptoms that fulfilled at least 4 of the American College of Rheumatology criteria for systemic LE. Symptoms manifested after a median duration of therapy of 4 months (etanercept) and 9 months (infliximab). After discontinuation of therapy, symptoms resolved either spontaneously or under topical or systemic therapy with glucocorticosteroids. No relapse of symptoms was observed. In some patients, skin lesions reminiscent of a chronic discoid LE were observed without detectable anti-DNA antibodies [36].

Elevated Liver Enzymes

Up to 8% of psoriasis patients treated with infliximab developed markedly elevated aspartate and alanine aminotransaminase levels (>150 U/l and ≥100% from baseline) [18], which was usually not associated with other indicators of liver function impairment. Treatment can be continued under close monitoring in most cases. However, severer hepatopathy may rarely occur (~3% of treated psoriasis patients) that usually resolves after discontinuation of the drug [17]. The following guidelines are used in clinical trials with respect to the elevation of aminotransferases: treatment possible with values <3 less than upper limit of normal (ULN); treatment with caution if values 3–5 above ULN; stop treatment if values >5 above ULN. Elevated liver enzymes have also been reported in patients treated with adalimumab, but less frequently (approx. 2–3% of patients with elevation of liver enzymes >2.5% of ULN), and discontinuations due to increases in liver enzymes or other laboratory abnormalities are rare [37, 38]. In a large study testing etanercept at different doses (25 mg/week, 25 mg twice weekly or 50 mg twice weekly for 24 weeks), only mild to moderate laboratory abnormalities were reported, and no patient discontinued therapy as a consequence of such abnormalities [39].

Serious Hematologic Events

TNF antagonists have rarely been associated with serious leukopenia, neutropenia, thrombocytopenia, pancytopenia or aplastic anemia. Rare lethal courses of aplastic anemia and pancytopenia in patients receiving etanercept occurred within a few weeks after initiation of therapy [40]. In 1 case report, mild neutropenia occurred after exposition to 2 different TNF antagonists, suggesting a class effect of TNF antagonists in this patient [41].

Malignancies

It remains controversial whether TNF antagonists are associated with a higher incidence of malignancies. TNF-α is involved in immunologic processes including tumor surveillance suggesting that (long-term) therapy with TNF antagonists might be associated with an increased risk of malignancies. On the other hand, disease activity in a number of diseases (such as rheumatoid arthritis and Crohn's disease) are associated with a higher tumor risk, so that it is conceivable that improved disease control achieved by anti-TNF therapy may also reduce the risk of developing malignancies.

From the data available so far, there is accumulating evidence for an increased risk of non-melanoma skin cancers, and probably also for melanoma, while data on other types of malignancies including lymphoma are much more inconsistent [42]. While several large observational studies have not shown an increased risk of cancer (excluding skin cancer) [42, 43], a meta-analysis of clinical trials with infliximab and adalimumab yielded a pooled odds ratio (OR) for malignancies of 2.02 (95% CI: 0.95–4.29) [44].

In psoriatic patients, a TNF-antagonist-associated risk of cutaneous malignancies might be particularly relevant, as many psoriatic patients have a history of therapy with cyclosporine and/or frequent UV-based therapies predisposing to a higher risk of developing cutaneous tumors. Therefore, inspection of skin should be performed regularly during and after treatment with TNF antagonists [45, 46].

The question of whether therapy with TNF antagonists leads to an increased risk of the rare and often fatal hepatosplenic T cell lymphoma has also not been answered yet. There are reports of the occurrence of this subtype of lymphoma in patients receiving infliximab or adalimumab [47]. These patients were mostly male adolescents or young adults suffering from inflammatory bowel disease, and on concurrent or prior therapy with azathioprine or 6-mercaptopurine, with the exception of a 61-year-old woman with rheumatoid arthritis and Felty syndrome. Although there are also reports on hepatosplenic T cell lymphomas in patients with inflammatory bowel disease receiving azathioprine or 6-mercaptopurine alone, a causal relationship with TNF antagonists cannot be excluded, and particularly an interaction between infliximab and azathioprine or 6-mercaptopurine and a potential genetic predisposition of patients with inflammatory bowel disease appears possible.

Overall, prolonged large prospective observational studies are needed to determine the long-term effects of TNF antagonists on the risk of malignancies, especially for malignancies with a low incidence rate. As the baseline risk differs between patients with different diseases, a separate evaluation is needed for TNF antagonists in the different indications.

Cardiovascular Events

It cannot be excluded that TNF antagonists induce or worsen chronic heart failure. In a review of data from European Biologic Registers [24], however, data neither indicated a TNF-antagonist-induced increased risk of new heart failure nor worsening of a preexisting heart failure. Furthermore, there was even a decrease in mortality from cardiovascular events in TNF-antagonist-treated patients compared to conventionally treated patients, with responders to TNF-antagonist therapy having a lower rate of myocardial infarctions than nonresponders.

Recommendations at present are that patients with well-compensated mild chronic heart failure of NYHA (New York Heart Association) classes I and II and an indication for the use of TNF antagonists should be evaluated at baseline and then be closely monitored for any clinical signs of worsening heart failure during therapy with TNF antagonists, while patients with NYHA class III or IV heart failure should not be treated with TNF antagonists.

Psoriasiform Dermatitis Induced or Worsened by TNF Antagonists

There are reports from more than 100 patients treated with TNF antagonists for indications other than psoriasis on manifestation of psoriasiform dermatitis or a pustular

Table 2. Characteristics of antibodies directed against TNF antagonists

	Infliximab [5, 17, 108–110]	Etanercept [52, 111]	Adalimumab [9, 112]
Frequency of anti-drug antibodies (approx. value), %	2–43	0–6	0.6–17
Neutralizing in vitro	yes	no	yes
Impact on efficacy	reduced long-term efficacy	no	titer-dependent decrease in efficacy
Impact on safety	increased risk of infusion reactions	no	no

Data are partly derived from the use of TNF antagonists in indications other than psoriasis.

variant of psoriasis [reviewed in 48]. In these cases, manifestation of psoriasis was not often accompanied by worsening of the disease for which TNF antagonists were applied. In patients suffering from plaque psoriasis, the manifestation of a pustular variant of psoriasis has also been reported in individual cases, both during and after cessation of therapy with TNF antagonists, and was accompanied by worsening of psoriasis in most cases [49]. In many cases, discontinuation of the current TNF antagonist is necessary, and initiation of another systemic therapy including a different TNF antagonist may be required.

Antibodies Directed against TNF Antagonists

TNF antagonists are not naturally occurring human proteins, and antibodies against these foreign proteins may develop (table 2). The exact frequency of formation of antidrug antibodies is not yet clear, and a comparison of studies is difficult as the methods used for detection have been improved lately and differ considerably. A higher proportion of patients develop antibodies to the chimeric antibody infliximab (approx. 2–43%) as compared to the fusion receptor protein etanercept (approx. 0–6%) or the human antibody adalimumab (approx. 0.6–17%).

However, the frequency depends on concomitant immunosuppressive therapy (lower in combination therapy with methotrexate), therapy duration and probably on the underlying disease. Antibodies to infliximab and adalimumab, but not to etanercept, have been shown to be neutralizing in vitro and to be associated with reduced treatment efficacy. There also seems to be a dose effect of antibodies to adalimumab on treatment efficacy, with higher concentrations being associated with a greater

TNF Antagonists in Other Forms of Psoriasis

TNF antagonists have been approved for plaque psoriasis and psoriatic arthritis, but not for other subtypes of psoriasis. However, case reports and small case series on the off-label use of TNF antagonists in these indications have been published. For example, in a case series of 10 patients with erythrodermic psoriasis receiving etanercept 25 mg twice weekly, 5 patients achieved a PASI 75 response after 12 weeks, and 6 patients had a PASI 75 response after 24 weeks [65]. In a series of 4 patients with recalcitrant erythrodermic psoriasis, infliximab at reduced doses between 2.7 and 4.4 mg/kg per infusion in combination with methotrexate led to an improvement in skin symptoms that could be maintained during the observation period (9 months to 5 years) [66]. Successful treatment of generalized pustular psoriasis has been reported for infliximab and adalimumab in several case reports, and in 1 case series of 4 patients [67–72]. In the latter case series, patients who had suffered a pustular flare of a preexisting chronic non-pustular psoriatic skin disease showed a rapid response to infliximab [69]. An increasing number of case reports also describe beneficial effects of TNF antagonists on localized palmoplantar pustular psoriasis. However, treatment of these subtypes of psoriasis with TNF antagonists represents an off-label therapy.

Special Aspects of Treatment Management and Patient Selection

Biologics are often used in patients with long-lasting or recalcitrant psoriasis, who require long-term systemic treatment. The selection and management of patients should ensure that drugs like TNF antagonists are used with a favorable risk/benefit profile for the patient. This process requires that physicians discuss risks, benefits and available alternatives with the patient, and that all patients undergo an assessment including the full clinical history, a thorough physical examination and further investigations with particular reference to the respective contraindications and toxicity profiles. Particularly in patients with relevant comorbidities, therapeutic decisions should be made using an interdisciplinary approach and therapy management should be tailored to the individual patient's needs.

As with other biologics, there is no evidence so far that TNF antagonists interfere with the metabolism or transport of other drugs; the cytochrome P450 system in particular is not affected. Therefore, there are no restrictions on combinations of TNF antagonists with other drugs based on pharmacokinetic drug-drug interactions.

It is mandatory to screen for active and latent tuberculosis before starting treatment with TNF antagonists, which should consist of a personal history of tuberculosis and a history of exposure to tuberculosis, a chest X-ray and a tuberculin skin test. Recommendations for testing procedures as well as algorithms for patients with inconclusive or positive test results vary between different countries. Recommendations for a Mendel-Mantoux skin test prior to treatment with TNF antagonists usually include a second 'booster' test on the contralateral arm in case of a weak reaction to the first skin test (induration ≤5 mm). In recent years, 2 novel tests for tuberculosis have become available, the QuantiFERON®-TB Gold test [73] and the ELISPOT-based T-Spot®-TB [74] both of which produce results within 24 h. They are not affected by prior bacille Calmette-Guérin vaccination or by infection with common non-tuberculous mycobacteria, and specificity appears to be superior to the Mendel-Mantoux skin test. While presently many national guidelines recommend the Mendel-Mantoux skin test for tuberculosis screening, the in vitro assays might eventually replace the Mendel-Mantoux skin test [75]. However, caution in the interpretation of the in vitro assays is particularly recommended in children and in immunosuppressed patients (as is also the case with the Mendel-Mantoux skin test) as there are still concerns about test sensitivity. If latent tuberculosis is suspected, TNF antagonist therapy may be initiated in combination with prophylactic treatment according to local guidelines, such as isoniazid, started 1 month before anti-TNF therapy and continued for 9 months. Presence of active tuberculosis is an absolute contraindication for therapy with any anti-TNF agent.

Further laboratory investigations before initiation of treatment with TNF antagonists should include a complete blood count, a differential white blood cell count, aspartate transaminase and alanine transaminase, as well as a urine pregnancy test according to German S3 guidelines [76]. However, a more extensive pretreatment screening may be considered. Routine laboratory parameters could include renal function test (creatinine, urea), serologic infection parameters (e.g. C-reactive protein) and urine analysis. Baseline values for ANA, ENA and anti-ds DNS antibodies might be helpful for comparison in case the development of a lupus-like syndrome is suspected during the course of therapy. In patients at increased risk, serology for hepatitis B and C (and probably HIV if the patient consents) should be performed. During therapy, routine laboratory analysis according to German S3 guidelines should consist of a complete blood count, a differential white blood cell count, aspartate transaminase and alanine transaminase, but probably a renal function test, urine analysis and C-reactive protein test could be added to this list.

For infliximab, monitoring of vital signs during and 1 h after the infusion is advisable, and infusions should be performed with immediate access to emergency treatment. Basic laboratory tests (clinical chemistry, blood count) are recommended before each infusion.

In addition, in patients at a particularly high risk of other diseases, e.g. oropharyngeal cancer in patients with a long-standing history of smoking and alcohol consumption, special investigations may be indicated to rule out the presence of such a disease or a precursor lesion before therapy.

As adverse events under therapy with TNF antagonists may have an insidious onset, an unusual presentation or take a rapid course, patient-reported symptoms may require earlier and more extensive investigations and therapeutic measures compared to patients without TNF antagonists or other immunosuppressive drugs.

It is important for physicians to assess the disease severity of psoriasis and the impact of the disease on the quality of life before and during treatment with TNF antagonists. If there is no significant improvement (e.g. no PASI 50 response) within 3 months of therapy with TNF antagonists, discontinuation of treatment should be considered.

Perioperative Management of TNF Antagonists

The question of whether to interrupt TNF antagonists around the time of elective surgery is frequently asked in the management of psoriasis patients. However, there are insufficient and inconclusive data from psoriasis patients and from patients using TNF antagonists for other indications [reviewed in 77]. For example, in a retrospective study of patients with rheumatoid arthritis undergoing orthopedic procedures, use of TNF antagonists was associated with the development of serious postoperative complications in a univariate analysis (OR: 4.4, 95% CI: 1.10–18.41, p = 0.041) and remained significant after controlling for other risk factors [78]. In contrast, in another retrospective study investigating surgical site infections, there was no increased risk from perioperative use of TNF antagonists (OR: 1.5, 95% CI: 0.43–5.2): However, crude infection rates were higher in patients in whom TNF antagonists were not interrupted at least 4 times the half-lives before the procedure (8.7%) compared to patients in whom TNF antagonists were interrupted at a later time point or were continued throughout the perioperative period (5.8%) and than in patients who did not receive TNF antagonists (4.0%) [79].

Due to the low frequency of serious perioperative infectious complications, the large variety of surgical interventions with different complication rates, the multitude of individual risk factors that have to be controlled for (e.g. comorbidities, age, comedication), a large number of patients would have to be enrolled in a prospective study to sufficiently address the question of perioperative management of TNF antagonists (and other immunosuppressive drugs), and therefore a prospective study is probably not going to be performed in the near future.

At present, there is no defined standard for perioperative care, neither for patients receiving TNF antagonists nor for patients using other DMARD. Ultimately, the risk of development of disease flares with the potential ensuing complications and reduction in physical and psychosocial well-being after interruption of TNF antagonists has to be weighed against a so far unknown perioperative risk of TNF antagonists. Particularly in large orthopedic surgical interventions, such as joint replacement surgery, infections of the joint prosthesis are associated with an increased mortality rate, and there is evidence that soft tissue and skin infections are increased in patients receiving TNF antagonists. As disease flares in psoriasis patients often develop with a time delay after discontinuation of systemic therapy, and the morbidity caused by a temporal interruption is usually limited in psoriasis patients and also in patients with psoriatic arthritis, a short-term interruption of systemic therapy usually does not cause serious damage. Therefore, in our centers, we usually recommend interrupting anti-TNF therapy before larger surgical interventions around 3–4 half-lives before the planned surgery, and initiate a consequent topical and/or UVB311 or PUVA therapy when the first signs of psoriasis reappear, particularly if the skin of the planned surgical site is involved.

TNF Antagonists in Overweight Patients

Psoriasis patients show an increased prevalence of obesity (BMI ≥30) and to be overweight (BMI 25–29). Increased BMI may affect the response to therapy in several ways, including indirect effects through differing endocrine and immune parameters between obese and normal-weight subjects such as increased TNF-α levels in obese subjects, and differences in drug dosage relative to body weight. In a subgroup analysis of 3 randomized trials with infliximab including 1,462 patients, PASI 75 responses after 10 weeks were comparable in patients with normal body weight (PASI 75: 77.5%), overweight patients (PASI75: 78.3%) and obese patients (PASI 75: 74.4%). In contrast, subgroup analyses of patients treated with etanercept in several studies suggest a reduced response rate (PASI 75 response) at week 12 in patients as stratified to BMI or to body weight [reviewed in 80]. For example, 25% of patients weighing more than 89.4 kg achieved a PASI 75 response at week 12, compared to 41% of patients weighing less than 89.4 kg. For adalimumab, no such subgroup analysis is available. In obese patients who do not respond to a TNF antagonist with a fixed dose, switching to a drug with a weight-adapted dose may be helpful.

TNF Antagonists in Patients on Hemodialysis

The elimination route(s) for the TNF antagonists have not been fully identified to date. Dose reduction in elderly patients does not seem to be necessary. Elimination in patients with kidney disease has not been studied. At present, there is no evidence that dose adjustment is necessary in patients with impaired renal function. In 6 patients with renal insufficiency, hemodialysis had no effect on etanercept serum concentrations, and etanercept kinetics were similar to the kinetics in psoriasis patients [81]. There are also case reports of 2 patients with rheumatoid arthritis on hemodialysis who were successfully treated with etanercept for at least 12 weeks [82, 83]. Experience with infliximab in patients on hemodialysis is limited to a few case reports. While treatment of 2 patients with rheumatoid arthritis was successful, infliximab used in patients with sarcoidosis and amyloidosis was accompanied by complications (hypercoagulate state and transient cytopenia associated with renal function impairment, respectively [reviewed in 84]). From the data available, cyclosporine can be used in psoriasis patients on hemodialysis without dose adjustment and cyclosporine blood concentrations can be monitored, so it probably is the systemic antipsoriatic drug of choice in psoriasis patients on hemodialysis. Although only limited data is available for etanercept, this TNF antagonist may be considered in cases where therapy with cyclosporine fails or is contraindicated and further systemic therapy is required.

TNF Antagonists in Patients Suffering from Hepatitis B/C or HIV Infection

Etanercept, when used as adjuvant therapy in addition to interferon α-2b and ribavirin in the treatment of chronic hepatitis C, has shown a significantly improved response compared to patients who received interferon α-2b and ribavirin without etanercept [85]. This suggests that etanercept (in combination with antiviral therapy) might be used in patients with chronic inflammatory disorders suffering from concomitant hepatitis C infection or in patients receiving interferon-α for therapy of hepatitis C who experience interferon-α-triggered exacerbation or a new onset of psoriasis. There are several case reports of the use of TNF antagonists for treatment of chronic inflammatory diseases, such as psoriasis in patients with hepatitis C, in whom no increase in liver enzymes and virus load was noted [86]. Patients with chronic viral hepatitis C receiving TNF antagonists should be appropriately evaluated and monitored during therapy with TNF antagonists. Data on the effect of TNF antagonists on chronic hepatitis B is very limited and mainly restricted to infliximab. Reactivation of chronic hepatitis B has been observed under therapy with infliximab in several cases [reviewed in 87]. Some case reports describe stable chronic hepatitis B in patients who receive co-treatment of infliximab and the antiviral nucleoside analogue lamivudine. However, in the absence of sufficient data, chronic carriers of hepatitis B should not be treated with TNF antagonists.

Treatment of psoriasis patients with HIV infection also poses a not infrequent therapeutic challenge, particularly as HIV infection can exacerbate psoriatic disease. There are several case reports on the use of etanercept and infliximab in patients with HIV infection and chronic inflammatory diseases, in whom no change in viral load was detected if determined [reviewed in 72], indicating that in patients with severe psoriasis and concomitant HIV infection and in whom no therapeutic alternative remains, therapy with TNF antagonists may be considered.

TNF Antagonists in Psoriatic Children

None of the TNF antagonists has been approved for the treatment of psoriasis in children. So far, a clinical trial with etanercept has been conducted in children between 4 and 17 years of age. Etanercept was used in a dosage of 0.8 mg/kg once weekly, up to a maximum dose of 50 mg/week; 57% of children in the treatment group compared to

11% in the placebo group achieved a PASI 75 response after 12 weeks, and the therapy was considered to be safe and effective [88]. Several case reports on the successful treatment of pediatric psoriasis patients with infliximab have also been published, with doses of 3.3 or 5 mg/kg at weeks 0, 2 and 6 and every 8 weeks thereafter [89, 90]. There are no published reports on the use of adalimumab in children suffering from psoriasis. On the other hand, there is more extensive experience with TNF antagonists in children from the use of TNF antagonists in other indications. Infliximab has been approved in children of at least 6 years of age in the indication Crohn's disease (first approval: 2006 by the FDA), etanercept in children 4 years or older in the indication juvenile idiopathic arthritis (first approval: 1999 by the FDA), and, in the USA, adalimumab in the same indication in children of at least 13 years of age (first approval: 2008 by the FDA).

Thus, there is evidence that TNF antagonists are effective in pediatric psoriatic patients, with most experience regarding etanercept. However, the use of TNF antagonists has to be carefully weighed against potential side effects. This is particularly important as the safety profile may differ between children and adults, and data to fully assess safety risk in children, particularly during long-term therapy, is insufficient.

Effects of TNF Antagonists on Comorbidities

Psoriasis patients have been found to suffer from increased metabolic and cardiovascular morbidity compared to the general population [91–93]. In particular, there was a significant association with cardiovascular death in patients with severe psoriatic disease and an early disease onset [94].

There is accumulating evidence that TNF antagonists might positively influence metabolic and cardiovascular parameters well established as risk factors for cardiovascular morbidity and mortality. For example, in patients with rheumatoid arthritis who achieved an ACR20 response over 1 year, carotid intima-media thickness had significantly decreased after 1 year of treatment with infliximab or etanercept, which was not the case in patients who had declined this therapy [95]. A significant improvement in insulin resistance from infliximab was found in patients with rheumatoid arthritis in a 14-week observational study on 19 patients [96], as well as in another study with a mean follow-up period of 9.6 months that included 9 patients [97]. In another study on 32 patients with rheumatoid arthritis treated with infliximab or etanercept, insulin sensitivity improved after 24 weeks of treatment (but not after 12 weeks of treatment), compared to no improvement in the control group of 20 patients receiving stable low-dose methotrexate or prednisolone [98].

The effect of TNF antagonists on the lipid profile is more controversial. In the majority of studies, no change in the atherogenic index (total cholesterol/HDL cholesterol) was found or such a change could not be maintained over a longer treatment period [99]. However, there are some indications of a possible favorable effect of TNF

16 Gottlieb AB, Evans R, Li S, Dooley LT, Guzzo CA, Baker D, Bala M, Marano CW, Menter A: Infliximab induction therapy for patients with severe plaque-type psoriasis: a randomized, double-blind, placebo-controlled trial. J Am Acad Dermatol 2004;51: 534–542.
17 Menter A, Feldman SR, Weinstein GD, Papp K, Evans R, Guzzo C, Li S, Dooley LT, Arnold C, Gottlieb AB: A randomized comparison of continuous vs. intermittent infliximab maintenance regimens over 1 year in the treatment of moderate-to-severe plaque psoriasis. J Am Acad Dermatol 2007;56:31.e1–e15.
18 Centocor: Prescribing information (Remicade 100 mg). Leiden, Centocor, April 2008.
19 Cheifetz A, Smedley M, Martin S, Reiter M, Leone G, Mayer L, Plevy S: The incidence and management of infusion reactions to infliximab: a large center experience. Am J Gastroenterol 2003;98:1315–1324.
20 Baert F, Noman M, Vermeire S, Van Assche G, D'Haens G, Carbonez A, Rutgeerts P: Influence of immunogenicity on the long-term efficacy of infliximab in Crohn's disease. N Engl J Med 2003;348:601–608.
21 Zeltser R, Valle L, Tanck C, Holyst MM, Ritchlin C, Gaspari AA: Clinical, histological, and immunophenotypic characteristics of injection site reactions associated with etanercept: a recombinant tumor necrosis factor alpha receptor: Fc fusion protein. Arch Dermatol 2001;137:893–899.
22 Mease PJ, Gladman DD, Ritchlin CT, Ruderman EM, Steinfeld SD, Choy EH, Sharp JT, Ory PA, Perdok RJ, Weinberg MA: Adalimumab for the treatment of patients with moderately to severely active psoriatic arthritis: results of a double-blind, randomized, placebo-controlled trial. Arthritis Rheum 2005; 52:3279–3289.
23 Gottlieb AB, Matheson RT, Lowe N, Krueger GG, Kang S, Goffe BS, Gaspari AA, Ling M, Weinstein GD, Nayak A, Gordon KB, Zitnik R: A randomized trial of etanercept as monotherapy for psoriasis. Arch Dermatol 2003;139:1627–1632.
24 Zink A, Askling J, Dixon WG, Klareskog L, Silman AJ, Symmons DP: European Biologics Registers – methodology, selected results, and perspectives. Ann Rheum Dis 2008, E-Pub ahead of print.
25 Bongartz T, Sutton AJ, Sweeting MJ, Buchan I, Matteson EL, Montori V: Anti-TNF antibody therapy in rheumatoid arthritis and the risk of serious infections and malignancies: systematic review and meta-analysis of rare harmful effects in randomized controlled trials. JAMA 2006;295:2275–2285.
26 Dixon WG, Watson K, Lunt M, Hyrich KL, Silman AJ, Symmons DP: Rates of serious infection, including site-specific and bacterial intracellular infection, in rheumatoid arthritis patients receiving anti-tumor necrosis factor therapy: results from the British Society for Rheumatology Biologics Register. Arthritis Rheum 2006;54:2368–2376.
27 Tubach F, Ravaud P, Salmon-Ceron D, Petitpain N, Brocq O, Grados F, Guillaume JC, Leport J, Roudaut A, Solau-Gervais E, Lemann M, Mariette X, Lortholary O: Emergence of *Legionella pneumophila* pneumonia in patients receiving tumor necrosis factor-alpha antagonists. Clin Infect Dis 2006;43: e95–e100.
28 Rychly DJ, DiPiro JT: Infections associated with tumor necrosis factor-alpha antagonists. Pharmacotherapy 2005;25:1181–1192.
29 Wallis RS, Broder M, Wong J, Lee A, Hoq L: Reactivation of latent granulomatous infections by infliximab. Clin Infect Dis 2005;41(suppl 3): S194–S198.
30 Winthrop KL: Risk and prevention of tuberculosis and other serious opportunistic infections associated with the inhibition of tumor necrosis factor. Nat Clin Pract Rheumatol 2006;2:602–610.
31 Gomez-Reino JJ, Carmona L, Angel DM: Risk of tuberculosis in patients treated with tumor necrosis factor antagonists due to incomplete prevention of reactivation of latent infection. Arthritis Rheum 2007;57:756–761.
32 Denis B, Lefort A, Flipo RM, Tubach F, Lemann M, Ravaud P, Salmon D, Mariette X, Lortholary O: Long-term follow-up of patients with tuberculosis as a complication of tumour necrosis factor (TNF)-alpha antagonist therapy: safe re-initiation of TNF-alpha blockers after appropriate anti-tuberculous treatment. Clin Microbiol Infect 2008;14:183–186.
33 Atzeni F, Sarzi-Puttini P, Dell' Acqua D, de Portu S, Cecchini G, Cruini C, Carrabba M, Meroni PL: Adalimumab clinical efficacy is associated with rheumatoid factor and anti-cyclic citrullinated peptide antibody titer reduction: a one-year prospective study. Arthritis Res Ther 2005;8:R3.
34 De Rycke L, Baeten D, Kruithof E, Van den Bosch F, Veys EM, De Keyser F: The effect of TNFalpha blockade on the antinuclear antibody profile in patients with chronic arthritis: biological and clinical implications. Lupus 2005;14:931–937.
35 De Bandt M, Sibilia J, Le Loët X, Prouzeau S, Fautrel B, Marcelli C, Boucquillard E, Siame JL, Mariette X, Club Rhumatismes et Inflammation: Systemic lupus erythematosus induced by anti-tumour necrosis factor alpha therapy: a French national survey. Arthritis Res Ther 2005;7:R545-R551.

36 Misery L, Perrot JL, Gentil-Perret A, Pallot-Prades B, Cambazard F, Alexandre C: Dermatological complications of etanercept therapy for rheumatoid arthritis. Br J Dermatol 2002;146:334–335.

37 Menter A, Tyring SK, Gordon K, Kimball AB, Leonardi CL, Langley RG, Strober BE, Kaul M, Gu Y, Okun M, Papp K: Adalimumab therapy for moderate to severe psoriasis: a randomized, controlled phase III trial. J Am Acad Dermatol 2008;58:106–115.

38 Gordon KB, Langley RG, Leonardi C, Toth D, Menter MA, Kang S, Heffernan M, Miller B, Hamlin R, Lim L, Zhong J, Hoffman R, Okun MM: Clinical response to adalimumab treatment in patients with moderate to severe psoriasis: double-blind, randomized controlled trial and open-label extension study. J Am Acad Dermatol 2006;55:598–606.

39 Leonardi CL, Powers JL, Matheson RT, Goffe BS, Zitnik R, Wang A, Gottlieb AB: Etanercept as monotherapy in patients with psoriasis. N Engl J Med 2003;349:2014–2022.

40 Phelan C, Wooltorton E: Infliximab and serious hematologic events. CMAJ 2004;171:1045.

41 Montane E, Salles M, Barriocanal A, Riera E, Costa J, Tena X: Antitumor necrosis factor-induced neutropenia: a case report with double positive rechallenges. Clin Rheumatol 2007;26:1527–1529.

42 Wolfe F, Michaud K: Biologic treatment of rheumatoid arthritis and the risk of malignancy: analyses from a large US observational study. Arthritis Rheum 2007;56:2886–2895.

43 Askling J, Fored CM, Brandt L, Baecklund E, Bertilsson L, Feltelius N, Coster L, Geborek P, Jacobsson LT, Lindblad S, Lysholm J, Rantapaa-Dahlqvist S, Saxne T, Klareskog L: Risks of solid cancers in patients with rheumatoid arthritis and after treatment with tumour necrosis factor antagonists. Ann Rheum Dis 2005;64:1421–1426.

44 Costenbader KH, Glass R, Cui J, Shadick N: Risk of serious infections and malignancies with anti-TNF antibody therapy in rheumatoid arthritis. JAMA 2006;296:2201–2204.

45 Marcil I, Stern RS: Squamous-cell cancer of the skin in patients given PUVA and ciclosporin: nested cohort crossover study. Lancet 2001;358:1042–1045.

46 Paul CF, Ho VC, McGeown C, Christophers E, Schmidtmann B, Guillaume JC, Lamarque V, Dubertret L: Risk of malignancies in psoriasis patients treated with cyclosporine: a 5 y cohort study. J Invest Dermatol 2003;120:211–216.

47 Drini M, Prichard PJ, Brown GJ, Macrae FA: Hepatosplenic T-cell lymphoma following infliximab therapy for Crohn's disease. Med J Aust 2008;189:464–465.

48 Wollina U, Hansel G, Koch A, Schonlebe J, Kostler E, Haroske G: Tumor necrosis factor-alpha inhibitor-induced psoriasis or psoriasiform exanthemata: first 120 cases from the literature including a series of six new patients. Am J Clin Dermatol 2008;9:1–14.

49 Mössner R, Thaci D, Mohr J, Patzold S, Bertsch HP, Krüger U, Reich K: Manifestation of palmoplantar pustulosis during or after infliximab therapy for plaque-type psoriasis: report on five cases. Arch Dermatol Res 2008;300:101–105.

50 Bartelds GM, Wijbrandts CA, Nurmohamed MT, Stapel S, Lems WF, Aarden L, Dijkmans BA, Tak PP, Wolbink GJ: Clinical response to adalimumab: relationship to anti-adalimumab antibodies and serum adalimumab concentrations in rheumatoid arthritis. Ann Rheum Dis 2007;66:921–926.

51 Skomsvoll JF, Wallenius M, Koksvik HS, Rodevand E, Salvesen KA, Spigset O, Kvien TK: Drug insight: anti-tumor necrosis factor therapy for inflammatory arthropathies during reproduction, pregnancy and lactation. Nat Clin Pract Rheumatol 2007;3:156–164.

52 Wyeth: Prescribing information (Enbrel 25 mg). Maidenhead, Wyeth, 2007.

53 Ostensen M, Eigenmann GO: Etanercept in breast milk. J Rheumatol 2004;31:1017–1018.

54 Mahadevan U, Terdiman JP, Aron J, Jacobsohn S, Turek P: Infliximab and semen quality in men with inflammatory bowel disease. Inflamm Bowel Dis 2005;11:395–399.

55 Zhou H: Clinical pharmacokinetics of etanercept: a fully humanized soluble recombinant tumor necrosis factor receptor fusion protein. J Clin Pharmacol 2005;45:490–497.

56 Felson DT, Anderson JJ, Boers M, Bombardier C, Furst D, Goldsmith C, Katz LM, Lightfoot R Jr, Paulus H, Strand V: American College of Rheumatology: preliminary definition of improvement in rheumatoid arthritis. Arthritis Rheum 1995;38:727–735.

57 Kavanaugh A, Antoni CE, Gladman DD, Wassenberg S, Zhou B, Beutler A, Keenan G, Burmester G, Furst DE, Weisman M, Kalden JR, Smolen J, van der HD: The Infliximab Multinational Psoriatic Arthritis Controlled Trial (IMPACT): results of radiographic analyses after 1 year. Ann Rheum Dis 2006;65:1038–1043.

58 van der Heijde D, Kavanaugh A, Gladman DD, Antoni C, Krueger GG, Guzzo C, Zhou B, Dooley LT, de Vlam K, Geusens P, Birbara C, Halter D, Beutler A: Infliximab inhibits progression of radiographic damage in patients with active psoriatic arthritis through one year of treatment: results from the induction and maintenance psoriatic arthritis clinical trial 2. Arthritis Rheum 2007;56:2698–2707.

59 Mease PJ, Kivitz AJ, Burch FX, Siegel EL, Cohen SB, Ory P, Salonen D, Rubenstein J, Sharp JT, Dunn M, Tsuji W: Continued inhibition of radiographic progression in patients with psoriatic arthritis following 2 years of treatment with etanercept. J Rheumatol 2006;33:712–721.

60 Mease PJ, Kivitz AJ, Burch FX, Siegel EL, Cohen SB, Ory P, Salonen D, Rubenstein J, Sharp JT, Tsuji W: Etanercept treatment of psoriatic arthritis: safety, efficacy, and effect on disease progression. Arthritis Rheum 2004;50:2264–2272.

61 Antoni C, Krueger GG, de Vlam K, Birbara C, Beutler A, Guzzo C, Zhou B, Dooley LT, Kavanaugh A: Infliximab improves signs and symptoms of psoriatic arthritis: results of the IMPACT 2 trial. Ann Rheum Dis 2005;64:1150–1157.

62 Antoni CE, Kavanaugh A, Kirkham B, Tutuncu Z, Burmester GR, Schneider U, Furst DE, Molitor J, Keystone E, Gladman D, Manger B, Wassenberg S, Weier R, Wallace DJ, Weisman MH, Kalden JR, Smolen J: Sustained benefits of infliximab therapy for dermatologic and articular manifestations of psoriatic arthritis: results from the infliximab multinational psoriatic arthritis controlled trial (IMPACT). Arthritis Rheum 2005;52:1227–1236.

63 Mease PJ, Goffe BS, Metz J, VanderStoep A, Finck B, Burge DJ: Etanercept in the treatment of psoriatic arthritis and psoriasis: a randomised trial. Lancet 2000;356:385–390.

64 Gladman DD, Mease PJ, Ritchlin CT, Choy EH, Sharp JT, Ory PA, Perdok RJ, Sasso EH: Adalimumab for long-term treatment of psoriatic arthritis: forty-eight week data from the adalimumab effectiveness in psoriatic arthritis trial. Arthritis Rheum 2007;56: 476–488.

65 Esposito M, Mazzotta A, de Felice C, Papoutsaki M, Chimenti S: Treatment of erythrodermic psoriasis with etanercept. Br J Dermatol 2006;155:156–159.

66 Heikkila H, Ranki A, Cajanus S, Karvonen SL: Infliximab combined with methotrexate as long-term treatment for erythrodermic psoriasis. Arch Dermatol 2005;141:1607–1610.

67 Schmick K, Grabbe J: Recalcitrant, generalized pustular psoriasis: rapid and lasting therapeutic response to antitumour necrosis factor-alpha antibody (infliximab). Br J Dermatol 2004;150:367.

68 Kamarashev J, Lor P, Forster A, Heinzerling L, Burg G, Nestle FO: Generalised pustular psoriasis induced by cyclosporin a withdrawal responding to the tumour necrosis factor alpha inhibitor etanercept. Dermatology 2002;205:213–216.

69 Trent JT, Kerdel FA: Successful treatment of Von Zumbusch pustular psoriasis with infliximab. J Cutan Med Surg 2004;8:224–228.

70 Benoit S, Toksoy A, Brocker EB, Gillitzer R, Goebeler M: Treatment of recalcitrant pustular psoriasis with infliximab: effective reduction of chemokine expression. Br J Dermatol 2004;150:1009–1012.

71 Callen JP, Jackson JH: Adalimumab effectively controlled recalcitrant generalized pustular psoriasis in an adolescent. J Dermatolog Treat 2005;16:350–352.

72 Mikhail M, Weinberg JM, Smith BL: Successful treatment with etanercept of von Zumbusch pustular psoriasis in a patient with human immunodeficiency virus. Arch Dermatol 2008;144:453–456.

73 Mazurek GH, Jereb J, Lobue P, Iademarco MF, Metchock B, Vernon A: Guidelines for using the QuantiFERON-TB Gold test for detecting *Mycobacterium tuberculosis* infection, United States. MMWR Recomm Rep 2005;54:49–55.

74 www.oxfordimmunotec.com/eu/products_services/tspottb.html (accessed January 9, 2009).

75 Beglinger C, Dudler J, Mottet C, Nicod L, Seibold F, Villiger PM, Zellweger JP: Screening for tuberculosis infection before the initiation of an anti-TNF-alpha therapy. Swiss Med Wkly 2007;137:620–622.

76 Nast A, Kopp IB, Augustin M, Banditt KB, Boehncke WH, Follmann M, Friedrich M, Huber M, Kahl C, Klaus J, Koza J, Kreiselmaier I, Mohr J, Mrowietz U, Ockenfels HM, Orzechowski HD, Prinz J, Reich K, Rosenbach T, Rosumeck S, Schlaeger M, Schmid-Ott G, Sebastian M, Streit V, Weberschock T, Rzany B: Evidence-based (S3) guidelines for the treatment of psoriasis vulgaris. J Dtsch Dermatol Ges 2007; 5(suppl 3):1–119.

77 Bongartz T: Elective orthopedic surgery and perioperative DMARD management: many questions, fewer answers, and some opinions.. J Rheumatol 2007;34:653–655.

78 Giles JT, Bartlett SJ, Gelber AC, Nanda S, Fontaine K, Ruffing V, Bathon JM: Tumor necrosis factor inhibitor therapy and risk of serious postoperative orthopedic infection in rheumatoid arthritis. Arthritis Rheum 2006;55:333–337.

79 den Broeder AA, Creemers MC, Fransen J, de JE, de Rooij DJ, Wymenga A, de Waal-Malefijt M, van den Hoogen FH: Risk factors for surgical site infections and other complications in elective surgery in patients with rheumatoid arthritis with special attention for anti-tumor necrosis factor: a large retrospective study. J Rheumatol 2007;34:689–695.

80 Clark L, Lebwohl M: The effect of weight on the efficacy of biologic therapy in patients with psoriasis. J Am Acad Dermatol 2008;58:443–446.

81 Don BR, Spin G, Nestorov I, Hutmacher M, Rose A, Kaysen GA: The pharmacokinetics of etanercept in patients with end-stage renal disease on haemodialysis. J Pharm Pharmacol 2005;57:1407–1413.

82 Sugioka Y, Inui K, Koike T: Use of etanercept in a patient with rheumatoid arthritis on hemodialysis. Mod Rheumatol 2008;18:293–295.

83 Cassano N, Vena GA: Etanercept treatment in a hemodialysis patient with severe cyclosporine-resistant psoriasis and hepatitis C virus infection. Int J Dermatol 2008;47:980–981.

84 Hammoudeh M: Infliximab treatment in a patient with rheumatoid arthritis on haemodialysis. Rheumatology (Oxford) 2006;45:357–359.

85 Zein NN: Etanercept as an adjuvant to interferon and ribavirin in treatment-naive patients with chronic hepatitis C virus infection: a phase 2 randomized, double-blind, placebo-controlled study. J Hepatol 2005;42:315–322.

86 Aslanidis S, Vassiliadis T, Pyrpasopoulou A, Douloumpakas I, Zamboulis C: Inhibition of TNFalpha does not induce viral reactivation in patients with chronic hepatitis C infection: two cases. Clin Rheumatol 2007;26:261–264.

87 Millonig G, Kern M, Ludwiczek O, Nachbaur K, Vogel W: Subfulminant hepatitis B after infliximab in Crohn's disease: need for HBV-screening? World J Gastroenterol 2006;12:974–976.

88 Paller AS, Siegfried EC, Langley RG, Gottlieb AB, Pariser D, Landells I, Hebert AA, Eichenfield LF, Patel V, Creamer K, Jahreis A: Etanercept treatment for children and adolescents with plaque psoriasis. N Engl J Med 2008;358:241–251.

89 Farnsworth NN, George SJ, Hsu S: Successful use of infliximab following a failed course of etanercept in a pediatric patient. Dermatol Online J 2005;11:11.

90 Menter MA, Cush JM: Successful treatment of pediatric psoriasis with infliximab. Pediatr Dermatol 2004;21:87–88.

91 Christophers E: Comorbidities in psoriasis. Clin Dermatol 2007;25:529–534.

92 Ludwig RJ, Herzog C, Rostock A, Ochsendorf FR, Zollner TM, Thaci D, Kaufmann R, Vogl TJ, Boehncke WH: Psoriasis: a possible risk factor for development of coronary artery calcification. Br J Dermatol 2007;156:271–276.

93 Boehncke S, Thaci D, Beschmann H, Ludwig RJ, Ackermann H, Badenhoop K, Boehncke WH: Psoriasis patients show signs of insulin resistance. Br J Dermatol 2007;157:1249–1251.

94 Mallbris L, Akre O, Granath F, Yin L, Lindelof B, Ekbom A, Stahle-Backdahl M: Increased risk for cardiovascular mortality in psoriasis inpatients but not in outpatients. Eur J Epidemiol 2004;19:225–230.

95 Del Porto F, Lagana B, Lai S, Nofroni I, Tinti F, Vitale M, Podesta E, Mitterhofer AP, D'Amelio R: Response to anti-tumour necrosis factor alpha blockade is associated with reduction of carotid intima-media thickness in patients with active rheumatoid arthritis. Rheumatology (Oxford) 2007;46: 1111–1115.

96 Tam LS, Tomlinson B, Chu TT, Li TK, Li EK: Impact of TNF inhibition on insulin resistance and lipids levels in patients with rheumatoid arthritis. Clin Rheumatol 2007;26:1495–1498.

97 Oguz FM, Oguz A, Uzunlulu M: The effect of infliximab treatment on insulin resistance in patients with rheumatoid arthritis. Acta Clin Belg 2007; 62:218–222.

98 Seriolo B, Paolino S, Ferrone C, Cutolo M: Effects of etanercept or infliximab treatment on lipid profile and insulin resistance in patients with refractory rheumatoid arthritis. Clin Rheumatol 2007;26:1799–1800.

99 Wijbrandts CA, van Leuven SI, Boom HD, Gerlag DM, Stroes ES, Kastelein JJ, Tak PP: Sustained changes in lipid profile and macrophage migration inhibitory factor (MIF) levels after anti-TNF therapy in rheumatoid arthritis. Ann Rheum Dis 2008, E-Pub ahead of print.

100 Popa C, van Tits LJ, Barrera P, Lemmers HL, van den Hoogen FH, van Riel PL, Radstake TR, Netea MG, Roest M, Stalenhoef AF: Anti-inflammatory therapy with TNF{alpha} inhibitors improves HDL-cholesterol anti-oxidative capacity in rheumatoid arthritis patients. Ann Rheum Dis, E-Pub ahead of print.

101 Krause D, Schleusser B, Herborn G, Rau R: Response to methotrexate treatment is associated with reduced mortality in patients with severe rheumatoid arthritis. Arthritis Rheum 2000;43:14–21.

102 Rich SJ: Considerations for assessing the cost of biologic agents in the treatment of psoriasis. J Manag Care Pharm 2004;10:S38–S41.

103 Sohn S, Schoeffski O, Prinz J, Reich K, Schubert E, Waldorf K, Augustin M: Cost of moderate to severe plaque psoriasis in Germany: a multicenter cost-of-illness study. Dermatology 2006;212:137–144.

104 Heinen-Kammerer T, Daniel D, Stratmann L, Rychlik R, Boehncke WH: Cost-effectiveness of psoriasis therapy with etanercept in Germany. J Dtsch Dermatol Ges 2007;5:762–768.

105 Papp KA, Tyring S, Lahfa M, Prinz J, Griffiths CE, Nakanishi AM, Zitnik R, van de Kerkhof PC, Melvin L: A global phase III randomized controlled trial of etanercept in psoriasis: safety, efficacy, and effect of dose reduction. Br J Dermatol 2005;152:1304–1312.

106 van de Kerkhof PC, Segaert S, Lahfa M, Luger TA, Karolyi Z, Kaszuba A, Leigheb G, Camacho FM, Forsea D, Zang C, Boussuge MP, Paolozzi L, Wajdula J: Once weekly administration of etanercept 50 mg is efficacious and well tolerated in patients with moderate-to-severe plaque psoriasis: a randomized controlled trial with open-label extension. Br J Dermatol 2008;159:1177–1185.
107 Tyring S, Gordon KB, Poulin Y, Langley RG, Gottlieb AB, Dunn M, Jahreis A: Long-term safety and efficacy of 50 mg of etanercept twice weekly in patients with psoriasis. Arch Dermatol 2007;143: 719–726.
108 Baraliakos X, Listing J, Rudwaleit M, Brandt J, Alten R, Burmester G, Gromnica-Ihle E, Haibel H, Schewe S, Schneider M, Sorensen H, Zeidler H, Visvanathan S, Sieper J, Braun J: Safety and efficacy of readministration of infliximab after long term continuous therapy and withdrawal in patients with ankylosing spondylitis. J Rheumatol 2007;34:510–515.
109 de Vries MK, Wolbink GJ, Stapel SO, de Vrieze H, Van Denderen JC, Dijkmans BA, Aarden LA, van der Horst-Bruinsma IE: Decreased clinical response to infliximab in ankylosing spondylitis is correlated with anti-infliximab formation. Ann Rheum Dis 2007;66:1252–1254.
110 Wolbink GJ, Vis M, Lems W, Voskuyl AE, de Groot E, Nurmohamed MT, Stapel S, Tak PP, Aarden L, Dijkmans B: Development of antiinfliximab antibodies and relationship to clinical response in patients with rheumatoid arthritis. Arthritis Rheum 2006;54:711–715.
111 de Vries MK, van der Horst-Bruinsma IE, Nurmohamed MT, Aarden LA, Stapel SO, Peters MJ, Van Denderen JC, Dijkmans BA, Wolbink GJ: Immunogenicity does not influence treatment with etanercept in patients with ankylosing spondylitis (AS). Ann Rheum Dis, E-pub ahead of print.
112 West RL, Zelinkova Z, Wolbink GJ, Kuipers EJ, Stokkers PC, Van der Woude CJ: Immunogenicity negatively influences the outcome of adalimumab treatment in Crohn's disease. Aliment Pharmacol Ther 2008;28:1122–1126.

Dr. Rotraut Mössner
Department of Dermatology, Georg August University
Von-Siebold-Strasse 3
DE–37075 Göttingen (Germany)
Tel. +49 551 396410, Fax +49 551 3922 047, E-Mail rmoessn@gwdg.de

Yawalkar N (ed): Management of Psoriasis.
Curr Probl Dermatol. Basel, Karger, 2009, vol 38, pp 137–159

Therapies for Childhood Psoriasis

Ralph M. Trüeb

Department of Dermatology, University Hospital of Zürich, Zürich, Switzerland

Abstract

With a prevalence of 2% of the general population of Europe and North America, psoriasis represents one of the most common and significant dermatologic disorders. While it has been claimed that psoriasis is uncommon in children, in fact 27% of cases manifest before the age of 16 years; moreover, psoriasis represents 4.1% of all dermatoses seen in children under the age of 16 years. Both recognition and treatment of psoriasis in children represent unique challenges. Early diagnosis and appropriate management are particularly important in children to lessen long-term disease-related psychosocial problems and comorbidities. Psoriasis in childhood is a disease of many forms, which may change over time. It may be difficult to recognize, since the frequencies of some types of patterns of psoriasis differ between adults and children, and some clinical features are distinctive to the pediatric age group. Management involves education of the child and parents concerning the nature of the disease and the effects of treatment. Environmental triggers should be sought and eliminated, particularly infection, trauma, and stress. The treatment options available are basically the same as for adults, but special care should be taken in order not to endanger the development or the future health of the child. In children, treatment modalities are limited because of safety concerns and/or poor compliance associated with messy and time-consuming therapies. Randomized controlled clinical trials involving children under the age of 12 years suffering from psoriasis have been reported only for 2 topical treatments, namely, calcipotriol and corticosteroids. Phototherapy and systemic therapy with methotrexate, acitretin and cyclosporin have limited use because of lower tolerability in children and cumulative toxicities. For this reason, treatments of psoriasis with the newer biologic agents, particularly the soluble tumor necrosis factor receptor fusion protein etanercept, are emerging. Finally, it is important to acknowledge that topical and systemic treatments are only part of a 'total care' package combining treatment, disease-specific education, and psychological support to cope with a possible lifelong skin condition.

Psoriasis is a chronic immune-mediated inflammatory disease most commonly manifested by well-demarcated erythematous silvery-scaled plaques on the elbows, knees, scalp and trunk. Psoriasis is probably one of the longest known illnesses of humans and, at least in the past, one of the most misunderstood. Some scholars believe psoriasis to have been included among the skin conditions called 'tzaraath' (Hebrew) in the

Bible (Leviticus chapters 13–14). The linguistic root of 'tzaraath' means 'smiting', in reference to a Talmudical explanation that it serves as a punishment for sin. It is quite possible that 'tzaraath' was a general term for certain types of skin disease, rather than a particular condition, and probably referred generally to any disease that produces eruptions on the skin. Later, psoriasis was frequently described as a variety of leprosy. The Greeks used the term 'lepra' (λεπρα) for scaly skin conditions, and the term 'psora' (ψωρα) to describe itchy skin conditions.

With an estimated prevalence of 1–3% worldwide, psoriasis represents one of the most common and significant skin disorders in dermatologic practice. Psoriasis affects both sexes equally and can occur at any age, although there are 2 peak incidences: approximately three quarters of patients develop their first lesions before the age of 40 years, with a first peak incidence between the ages of 16 and 21 years; the disease manifests in the other quarter of patients at a second peak incidence in the sixth decade of life [1]. For years it has been stated that psoriasis is uncommon in childhood. Yet, the Stanford Psoriasis Life History Survey of 5,600 adult psoriatic patients disclosed that 27% of patients reported an onset of psoriasis before the age of 16 years, 10% before age 10 years, 6.5% before age 5 years, and 2% before age 2 years [2]. Moreover, psoriasis represents 4.1% of all dermatoses seen in children under the age of 16 years in Europe and North America [3]. In both childhood and adolescence, psoriasis has been reported to be more common in girls than in boys, with a female-to-male ratio of 2:1, and seems to start at a younger age in girls. A recently published clinical review of 1,262 cases of childhood psoriasis in children between 1 month and 15 years of age, underlines the significance of childhood psoriasis, its clinical particularities, and therapeutic challenges [4].

Genetic Background

A genetic background has been suggested by the observation of a positive family history in patients with psoriasis. Evidence of family history of psoriasis has been documented in several large studies, ranging from 10 to over 70% [5, 6], and appears to be more common among children than adult patients [4]. A study on first-degree relatives of 3,095 psoriatic patients found a life-time risk of psoriasis with no parent, 1 parent, or both parents with psoriasis to be 4, 28, and 65%, respectively [5]. The risk was found to be higher if there was already 1 child with psoriasis in the family. Also, the risk of psoriasis arising before the age of 32 years was found to correlate with the age of onset of psoriasis in the parent(s) [5].

Interestingly, a higher prevalence of psoriasis has been suggested for Turner's syndrome (17%) [7].

Finally, through twin studies, a role for environmental factors in the development of disease has also been suggested, since a monozygotic twin concordance of 35% and a dizygotic twin concordance of 12% has been shown in 1 study [8].

Environmental Triggers

Precipitation of psoriasis by environmental factors is well documented for: group A β-hemolytic streptococcal infections [9, 10], trauma [11] and stress [12]. Human immunodeficiency virus infection has been reported in association with widespread psoriasis (also in infants) [13, 14], *Pityrosporum ovale* folliculitis with guttate psoriasis [15], and *Candida albicans* infection with psoriatic exacerbation and persistence [16]. As in adults, some drugs have been reported to induce or exacerbate psoriasis in children, such as growth hormone, lithium, β-blocking agents, and recombinant γ- and α-interferon.

Group A β-hemolytic streptococcal infections typically induce psoriasis of the guttate type, but pustular childhood psoriasis has also been reported to be elicited by streptococcal infection [10]. Both throat infection and perianal streptococcal disease have been documented prior to the onset of guttate psoriasis in children [17]. The process by which psoriatic flares occur in susceptible individuals after group A β-hemolytic streptococcal infections has been proposed to be two-fold. Streptococcal superantigen activates CD4+ T cells, and a large percentage of these home to the skin as the target organ. Once there, they liberate cytokines that attract CD8+ lymphocytes, which induce susceptible transient amplifying cells. A burst of mitotic activity occurs, inducing the early lesions of psoriasis. The hyperproliferative psoriatic epidermis increases the expression of keratins, such as keratin 14. This cycle may be perpetuated by T cells sensitized specifically to streptococcal M protein, which shares a striking homology with keratin 14 in the skin [18]. Association of psoriatic eruptions with Kawasaki disease might be in favor of the superantigen theory [19].

Patterns of Clinical Presentation

On the basis of age of onset, family history and associated genetic markers, a distinction has been proposed: (1) type I psoriasis, with an early onset (before 40 years), positive family history, and association with HLA-Cw6, -B57, and -DR7; (2) type II psoriasis, with late onset (after 40 years), negative family history, and association with HLA-Cw2 [20]. Patients with early onset psoriasis (type I) tend to have severer disease, with large body coverage and frequent recurrences, while late-onset psoriasis (type II) tends to be more localized and stable. Although, by definition, childhood psoriasis is type I psoriasis, early onset of childhood psoriasis does not necessarily correlate with a more serious prognosis.

The clinical presentations of childhood psoriasis are varied, with age-related peculiarities [16].

Congenital and Infantile Psoriasis

In a study reviewing 1,262 cases of childhood psoriasis in Australia, 16% of the subjects were less than 1 year and 27% less than 2 years of age [4]. The most frequent manifestation of psoriasis in these age groups was psoriatic diaper rash with dissemination.

Psoriatic Erythroderma

Rarely, psoriasis can be congenital, sometimes presenting as a nonspecific erythroderma (fig. 1). Psoriasis was the etiology of erythroderma in the first year of 4% of 51 infants from a reported case series [21]. Clinically, scalp hyperkeratosis and nail involvement favor the diagnosis.

Psoriatic Diaper Rashes

Psoriatic rashes in the diaper distribution present in 2 distinctive appearances: localized psoriatic diaper rash, and psoriatic diaper rash with dissemination. Some children may only ever have the characteristic well-demarcated bright-red rash localized exclusively to the diaper area (fig. 2), while others have this rash as an apparent first stage, later progressing, often explosively, to psoriatic diaper rash with dissemination. Differential diagnosis of localized psoriatic diaper rash from seborrheic dermatitis, irritant contact dermatitis and *Candida albicans* infection may be difficult. Moreover, the irritant contact dermatitis induced by the nappy, as well as infection by *Candida albicans*, may induce Koebner phenomenon allowing a psoriatic diathesis to express itself. More sharply demarcated lesions, a positive family history, the presence of other suggestive lesions, or the presence of nail pits favor the diagnosis of psoriasis. In some cases, a definitive diagnosis will be made only over the course of time.

Childhood and Adolescence Psoriasis

Psoriasis in childhood and adolescence is in many ways similar to adulthood. As in adults, classical plaque psoriasis represents the most frequent clinical form in children. Due to a number of factors, some children may present with rashes that show features of both eczema and psoriasis (eczema-psoriasis overlap), at times making the differential diagnosis difficult [4]. During childhood and adolescence, the initial manifestation of psoriasis is often triggered through an infection. The typical presentation in these cases is guttate psoriasis.

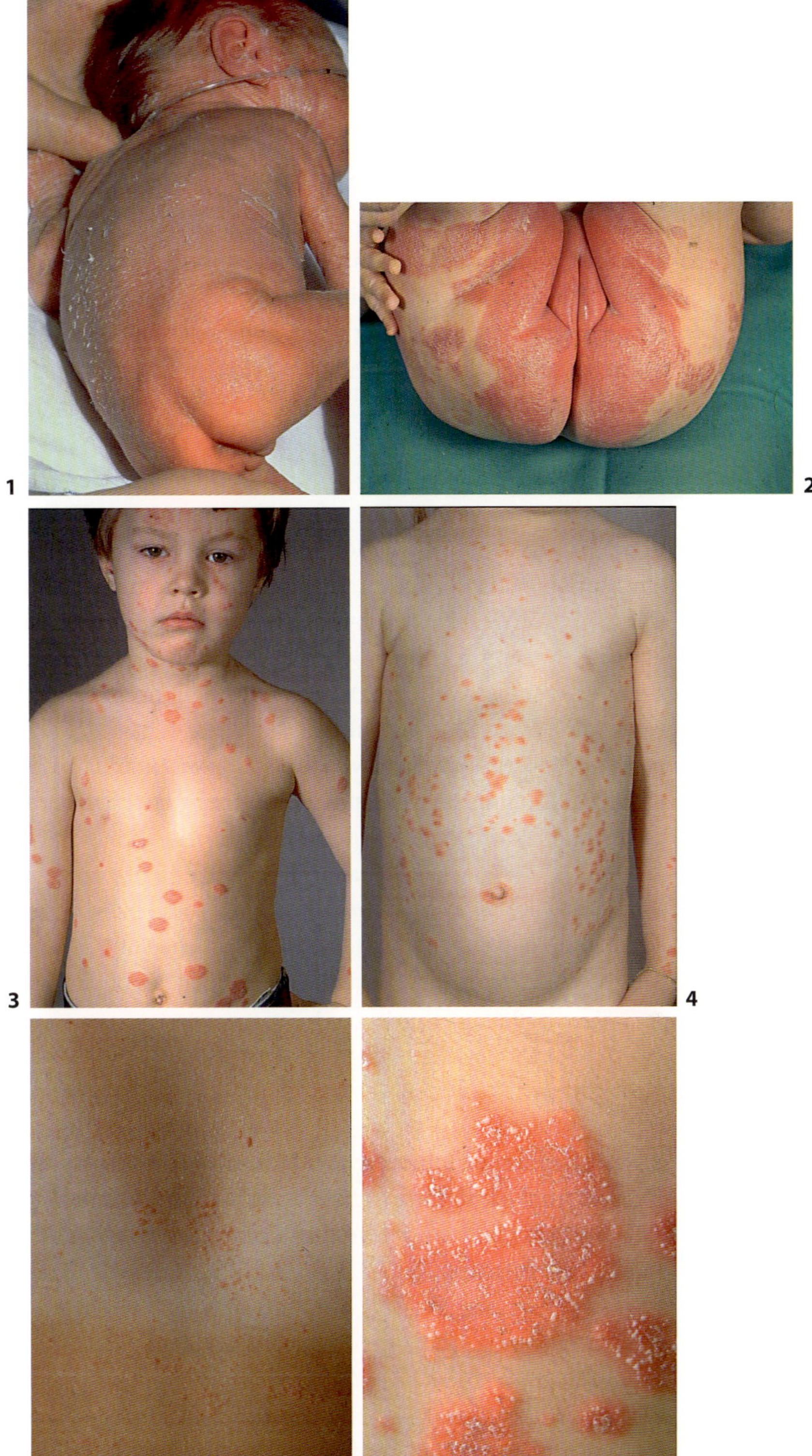

Fig. 1. Congenital erythroderma.
Fig. 2. Psoriatic diaper rash.

Fig. 3. Plaque psoriasis.
Fig. 4. Acute guttate psoriasis.

Fig. 5. Micropapular psoriasis.
Fig. 6. Subacute annular pustular psoriasis.

Plaque Psoriasis

Psoriasis in children may present in the typical adult form of large erythematous plaques, with a thick silver-white scale, predominantly on the extensor surfaces, knees, buttocks, elbows, and scalp. Usually, however, in children the plaques tend to be smaller and the scale is finer (fig. 3). Even large plaques of psoriasis in children have a scale that is softer and finer than is usual in psoriatic plaques in adults. In dark-skinned children, the scale may be so subtle that the condition presents as hypopigmentation, and the scale becomes obvious only when the lesions are scratched. Occurrence of the plaque form in children with psoriasis has been reported with frequencies between 34% [4] and 84% [22].

Acute Guttate Psoriasis

Another common presentation of psoriasis in children is acute guttate psoriasis with an eruption of small papules in a widespread distribution (fig. 4). The exanthematous eruption is often preceded by an intercurrent illness, usually a pharyngitis or tonsillitis due to group A β-hemolytic streptococci. It may also be precipitated by perianal streptococcal disease, which is why swabbing of both the pharynx and perianal area is recommended in these patients [17]. In a retrospective study of 245 patients with psoriasis, exacerbation following tonsillitis was noted in 133 (54%), usually within 2–3 weeks of infection [23]. Streptococci were isolated from throat swabs in 33 out of 34 patients (97%) [24], and serologic evidence of streptococcal infection was demonstrated in 56–85% [24–26]. The initial presentation of guttate psoriasis is quite monomorphic, later it may evolve into plaque psoriasis or completely resolve within 3–4 months after elimination of exacerbating factors. Occurrence of the acute guttate form in children with psoriasis has been reported with frequencies of between 6.4 and 44% [4, 22, 27].

Micropapular Psoriasis

A micropapular or follicular form of psoriasis occurs with 1- to 2-mm papules (fig. 5), most marked on the extensor aspects of the limbs. They are found particularly in dark-skinned children, where they usually are skin-colored, until scratching demonstrates the white scale.

Facial Involvement

Psoriatic involvement of the face is more common in children than in adults, and was found in 38% of children with psoriasis in the Australian case series [4]. It presents with erythematous, well-defined, and often symmetrical lesions on the cheeks. A common site is under the eyes. Lesions are characteristically more clearly demarcated than eczematous patches, are less itchy, and quite often have an annular configuration. Facial involvement is difficult to ascribe to psoriasis when it is the only presenting manifestation. Facial psoriasis was the sole manifestation of psoriasis in 4% of the Australian study [4].

Scalp Psoriasis

The scalp is a common site of disease involvement at the onset and throughout the course of psoriasis. Scalp psoriasis and its pityriasis amiantacea variant may be associated with the various forms of psoriasis or they may be isolated findings. The clinical presentation is highly variable, ranging from mild disease, with slight fine scaling, to severe disease, with thick crusted plaques covering the entire scalp. The back of the head is a common site, but multiple discrete areas of the scalp or the whole scalp may be affected. Scalp psoriasis is characterized by thick silvery white scale on patches of erythema. It may extend beyond the hairline. Even though often covered by the hair, scalp psoriasis is often a source of embarrassment due to flaking of the scale. Moreover, scalp psoriasis may be extremely itchy.

Pityriasis amiantacea is a condition of the scalp characterized by thick yellow-white scales densely coating the scalp skin and adhering to the scalp hairs as they exit the scalp. They are arranged in an overlapping manner like flakes of asbestos, hence the name. Depending on the underlying disorder, the scalp skin may appear normal, or may be deeply erythematous. Pityriasis amiantacea usually affects only part of the scalp, but may occasionally involve the whole scalp. Some hair loss is common in areas of pityriasis amiantacea, but hair regrows normally if the condition is effectively treated. This hair loss is sometimes aggravated by the difficulty in combing the hair due to the adherent thick scale at the base of hair shafts. If additional complications such as secondary bacterial infection occur, hair loss may be associated with scarring and then be permanent (psoriatic scarring alopecia). Pityriasis amiantacea may be present without any obvious underlying cause, but may be associated with psoriasis or other dermatologic conditions. Scalp ringworm (tinea capitis) is an important differential diagnosis, especially in children.

Inverse, Flexural or Intertriginous Psoriasis

Inverse psoriasis is located on genital, perianal, axillary, inguinal, or periumbilical areas. Localization in the labial folds or interdigital toe webs may pose special differential diagnostic problems. Inverse psoriasis usually appears as well-demarcated glazed erythematous lesions lacking the psoriatic scale. Local factors, such as maceration, bacterial (streptococcal) or fungal infections *(Candida albicans)*, may modify or aggravate psoriasis in these locations. In the Australian childhood psoriasis case series, it occurred with a frequency of 8.9% [4].

Palmoplantar Psoriasis

Psoriasis of the palm and sole varies in appearance, from thick scaling with fissuring to a glazed erythema. A common feature is a clear cutoff at the wrist fold. Palmoplantar psoriasis occurred in approximately 4% of patients in several pediatric psoriasis series [4, 22].

Psoriasiform/Psoriatic Acral Dermatitis

This peculiar clinical presentation of psoriasis was first described by Zaias [28] in 1980. It is characterized by cutaneous involvement of the digits without the typical nail dystrophy of psoriasis. Features are erythema, scales, and fissures of the distal phalanges associated with a remarkable shortening of the nail bed. Psoriasiform acral dermatitis may be isolated or associated with typical lesions of psoriasis in other areas, and therefore the most appropriate term to define it has been proposed to be 'psoriatic acral dermatitis' [29].

Nail Involvement

Psoriatic changes have been reported in 7–40% of children younger than 18 years of age [30], and may be an isolated finding or associated with the different forms of psoriasis. In one study, nail pitting was the most common nail change at 87%, followed by onycholysis in 10%, longitudinal striations and subungual hyperkeratosis in 8% each, and nail discoloration in 5%; in 2%, nail pitting alone was the first sign of the disease [31]. Besides these changes, trachyonychia (20 nail dystrophy) is found in childhood psoriasis. Nail changes may also be seen among psoriatic arthritis patients, with pitting and longitudinal striations being most frequent [32].

Pustular Psoriasis

Pustular psoriasis is rare and occurs more frequently in the adult population. Four forms have been described: generalized pustular psoriasis (von Zumbusch), subacute annular pustular psoriasis (Lapière), palmoplantar pustular psoriasis and pustular acrodermatitis of Hallopeau. Mixed variants are also possible.

The subacute annular form or recurrent circinate erythematous psoriasis of Lapière is the most frequent form in children, and is characterized by annular plaques with a pustular margin (fig. 6) [33].

Generalized pustular psoriasis of the von Zumbusch type is an acute erythroderma with diffuse pustules all over the body surface. Systemic toxicity and high fevers may occur. Often, the condition will resolve spontaneously in several weeks, leaving normal skin. Recurrence is common and usually occurs with a more typical psoriatic plaque presentation. Streptococcal infection has been described as a possible triggering factor [10].

Localized pustular psoriasis of the palms and soles (acropustulosis) has been noted to occur rarely in children [19]. Palmoplantar pustular psoriasis is often symmetrical with pinhead pustules that may coalesce, while the pustular acrodermatitis of Hallopeau involves only a few fingers with possible destruction of the distal phalanx and nail organ. In the Australian case series, acropustulosis was found in 4.7% of childhood psoriasis cases; 68% of acropustulosis cases occurred in children less than 5 years of age [4].

Mucosal Involvement

Psoriasis-related mucosal lesions were seen in 5.6% of children with psoriasis in one study [31]. Lesions included erythematous mucosal patches on oral or genital mucosae (psoriatic vulvitis, psoriatic balanitis), oral erosions, and geographic tongue (exfoliatio linguae areata). While it is not common for the latter condition to cause pain, it may cause a burning or stinging sensation after contact with certain foods, such as spicy or citrus foods.

Psoriatic Arthropathy

Psoriatic arthropathy is a rare condition in children. The peak age of onset is 9–12 years, and there is a slight female:male predominance of 3:2 [16]. The clinical presentations and course are similar to adults, but pediatric psoriatic arthritis may be difficult to diagnose because of similarities in clinical presentation with juvenile rheumatoid arthritis. In general, skin lesions precede the onset of psoriatic arthritis in 80% of patients. The following diagnostic criteria for psoriatic arthropathy in children have been proposed by the International League Against Rheumatism [34]:

1 Arthritis and psoriasis, or
2 Arthritis and
   a a family history of medically confirmed psoriasis in parents or siblings;
   b dactylitis;
   c nail abnormalities (pitting or onycholysis).

Exclusions:

a positive rheumatoid test;

b presence of systemic arthritis.

Distinct manifestations of psoriatic arthropathy based on the chronicity of disease exist: oligoarthritis (involving the proximal and distal interphalangeal joints of the feet, proximal interphalangeal joints of the hand, as well as the knees and ankles) is commonly seen during the early stages. Over time, polyarthritis may develop to include the wrist, metacarpophalangeal, elbow, and metatarsophalangeal joints. A distinguishing feature also sometimes found is blue discoloration over affected joints. Paying attention to spinal involvement can also be helpful in diagnosing psoriatic arthropathy and, in rare cases, other systemic manifestations such as uveitis and inflammatory bowel disease have been noted in both adults and children [30].

The course of childhood psoriatic arthropathy is unpredictable, with successive remissions and relapses. In most patients, the prognosis is good with minimal or absent joint disease in adulthood. In severe cases, however, psoriatic arthropathy may be rapidly progressive and incapacitating, producing destruction of the joints (psoriasis mutilans) [16].

In the recent past, distinctive entities affecting the skin and bones related to psoriasis have been recognized: pustulotic arthroosteitis (Sonosaki et al. [35]), chronic recurrent multifocal osteomyelitis, SAPHO syndrome, and psoriatic onycho-pachydermo periostitis [36].

The acronym SAPHO (synovitis, acne, pustulosis, hyperostosis, osteitis) has been coined to emphasize the association between osteoarticular inflammation and aseptic neutrophilic dermatologic disorders, including psoriasis. Chronic recurrent multifocal osteomyelitis is a manifestation of SAPHO syndrome in adults. Pediatric cases of SAPHO syndrome have been reported [37]. The associated dermatologic conditions were most often variants of psoriasis, with palmoplantar pustular psoriasis occurring in 56%, non-palmoplantar pustular psoriasis in 8%, and non-pustular psoriasis in 22%. Pustulotic arthroosteitis, as originally described by Sonosaki et al. [35] in 1981, is an association of palmoplantar pustulosis with sternoclavicular osteoarthritis, and is probably a manifestation of the SAPHO syndrome.

Psoriatic onycho-pachydermo periostitis presents with painful enlargement and nail deformity of the great toes [38, 39]. Patients present with nail changes, usually onycholysis and longitudinal striation, in association with underlying bone pathology (condensation, periosteal proliferation), and painful soft tissue swelling [38, 39]. The condition has to be differentiated from pustular acrodermatitis of Hallopeau, and does not involve the distal interphalangeal joints. The condition has so far only been reported in adults.

Therapy

As delineated in the first section of this chapter, childhood psoriasis is a disease of many forms that may change over time. It may be difficult to recognize, since the frequencies of some types of patterns of psoriasis differ between adults and children, and some clinical features are distinctive to the pediatric age group. Early diagnosis and appropriate management are particularly important in children to lessen long-term disease-related psychosocial problems and comorbidities.

The treatment options available for children are basically the same as for adults; however, children are not simply small adults. The treatment of psoriasis in all age groups has developed largely empirically, and there are few comparative trials in children. Randomized controlled clinical trials involving children under the age of 12 years suffering from psoriasis have been reported only for 2 topical treatments, namely, calcipotriol and corticosteroids. The use of other antipsoriatic treatments in children is based on adult psoriasis studies, case reports, retrospective analysis, open studies, and personal experience of pediatric dermatologists.

In children, treatment modalities are limited because of safety concerns and/or poor compliance associated with messy and time-consuming therapies.

When treating pediatric psoriasis, special care should be taken in order not to endanger the development or the future health of the child. Peculiarities of pharmacotherapy in children are: (1) a higher penetration of pharmacologic agents through the skin with a bigger risk of resorptive toxicities [children are especially susceptible to agents that may have a negative influence on growth and development, such as corticosteroids, vitamin D analogues, retinoids, and methotrexate (MTX)]; (2) age-dependent variations in the efficacy and safety of pharmacologic agents, due to differences in metabolization, penetration, distribution, and drug elimination kinetics. Dosage recommendations are usually given in relation to age, though the body weight and surface are relevant. In infants, dosage is chosen according to the body weight and in older children according to the body surface, extrapolated from the body height and weight using nomograms. In general, 6- to 9-year-old children are treated with half the adult dose, and children of 10–12 years with two thirds of the dose.

Finally, it should be remembered that in young children compliance is dependent almost entirely on the parents. Education of the child and parents concerning the nature of psoriasis is especially important to encourage a positive approach to the condition and its treatment. Through the school years and adolescence, considerable support is needed to cope with the reactions of other children to the disease. The concept of total care [40, 41] encompasses treating and addressing the visible, social, and psychological aspects associated with the disease. Ideally, treating all facets of psoriasis in children will result in a more motivated and understanding patient and parents, and improved compliance leading to more frequent and prolonged remission periods. Total care includes:

- developing a close parent-child-physician relationship;
- educating both the parents and the child;
- identifying, preventing, and/or treating precipitating factors such as infections, stress, trauma, or sunburns;
- selecting tonsillectomy and adenoidectomy in cases of recurrent throat infections;
- developing self-esteem and providing psychological support;
- providing access to support groups;
- maintaining a wellness program, including exercise and diet to maintain an ideal weight;
- providing access to a multidisciplinary team if required (otorhinolaryngology, rheumatology, psychology, social work);
- maintaining adequate skin care.

Early treatment and education can reduce later complications [41].

Elimination of Exacerbating Factors

The environmental triggers of psoriasis are different from those in adults: children take less drugs and alcohol, but are more exposed to trauma and infections. It has also been suggested that early-onset psoriasis is more frequently exacerbated by stress than late-onset psoriasis [23]. Accordingly, treatment of psoriasis also aims to eliminate exacerbating factors, e.g. there is a strong association between streptococcal pharyngitis and the activity of psoriasis, especially acute guttate psoriasis. Also, it should be remembered that perianal streptococcal dermatitis may be another site of infection. There is anecdotal evidence that treating infection improves psoriasis, particularly acute guttate psoriasis, for which prophylactic antibiotics (penicillin, erythromycin) or tonsillectomy have been advocated [42]. However, there are no controlled trials.

Topical Therapy

Most children with psoriasis are managed with topical treatment. Treatment must be prudent. The most commonly used topical medications include salicylic acid, topical corticosteroids, coal tar, anthralin, and calcipotriol.

Mild emollients such as petrolatum can be used in all age groups. During pre-adolescent years and older, emollients with keratolytics may be considered. Care must be taken to avoid overuse of salicylic-acid-containing topicals, as this practice can lead to salicylate intoxication. Symptoms are those of acidemia, central nervous system depression (ranging from somnolence and lethargy to seizures and coma), and renal failure. We prefer using bland emollients, such as unguentum emulsificans aquosum, to which 5% urea may be added. In mild psoriasis, the regular use of emollients and frequent sunbathing, with avoidance of overexposure, may be sufficient.

Topical Corticosteroids

Topical corticosteroids are the most popular treatment for psoriasis. Many of them have been studied in children with atopic dermatitis, but not psoriasis. A large array of potencies and delivery forms are available, although only few have pediatric usage listed as an approved indication on the drug label. Approved steroidal therapies for treatment of psoriasis in children are mometasone furoate and alclometasone dipropionate. Long-term use or the use of higher-potency topical corticosteroids should be avoided or used sparingly in children. The adverse effects of topical corticosteroids include atrophy, striae, hypothalamic-pituitary-adrenal (HPA) axis suppression, and tachyphylaxis. Children may be more susceptible to HPA axis suppression resulting from their increased surface-to-body mass ratio.

For the facial area, diaper area, and intertriginous lesions, mild corticosteroids such as 1% hydrocortisone are preferred, since these areas are particular susceptible to the adverse effects of topical corticosteroids.

Coal Tar

Topical coal tar or liquor carbonis detergens has been prescribed for the treatment of psoriasis for many years and has been shown to be particularly effective when used in combination with UVB light (Goeckerman regimen). It has anti-inflammatory, antipruritic and antimitotic effects. Liquor carbonis detergens has been helpful in all age groups, but in older children the smell limits its suitability. The short-term side effects are folliculitis, irritation, contact allergy, and phototoxicity. Irritancy is a special concern in infants, as it may occur at any age when applied to the face or intertriginous areas. Due to the high polycyclic aromatic hydrocarbon content of tars, concern has arisen with respect to carcinogenicity. The carcinogenicity of coal tar has been shown in animal studies and studies in occupational settings. Currently, coal tar is predominantly used in 1–5% shampoo formulations for treatment of scalp psoriasis. Dermal uptake of polycyclic aromatic hydrocarbons after hair washing with coal tar (after single treatment: 0.4–8.3 μmol per mol creatinine) are comparable to values in coke oven workers, and biotransformation to reactive metabolites in human hair follicles have been shown. However, studies of patients with psoriasis who are treated with coal tar do not indicate an increased incidence of skin cancer or internal tumors.

Anthralin

Anthralin or dithranol is a hydroxyanthrone, anthracene derivative, which has been in use as a antipsoriatic treatment for over 100 years. It is available as creams, ointment, or pastes in 0.1–2% concentrations. Anthralin accumulates in mitochondria where it interferes with the supply of energy to the cell, probably by the oxidation of anthralin-releasing free radicals. This impedes DNA replication and slows down the excessive cell division that occurs in psoriatic plaques. More anthralin penetrates into impaired skin in 30 min than into intact skin during about 16 h. For this reason, weaker 0.1–0.5% preparations are applied overnight, but stronger 1–2% products are

Phototherapy

Phototherapy involves exposing the skin to wavelengths of UV light under medical supervision. The ability of sunlight to lessen the severity of psoriasis has been known for a long time, and is the basis of heliotherapy (sunbathing). The biblical story of the prophet Elisha who heals the Syrian Captain Naeman (2 Kings 5) probably represents an early form of balneo-phototherapy, the combination of bathing and UV exposure. When patients have psoriasis that does not respond to topical medications alone or lesions that are too extensive for topical treatment, phototherapy becomes an option. Both outpatient and home light box therapy are available, depending on the needs and responsibility of the patient and caregivers.

Ultraviolet B

UVB has been demonstrated to be a safe and efficacious treatment for psoriasis, and has been used for years by dermatologists. Its most important adverse effect is temporary erythema. Narrowband UVB (311 nm) has been shown to clear plaques at a lesser, more suberythodermic, dose than broadband UVB [51]. In the absence of any clear evidence concerning the long-term safety of UVB, divergent opinions have been expressed as to the role of UVB phototherapy in children. Parents are probably better advised that there may be a slight increase in photoaging and risk of skin cancer. UVB occasionally exacerbates acute guttate psoriasis. For young children, a caregiver may need to accompany the child into the light box in order to help avert fear and to prevent the contact with hot light bulbs or removal of safety glasses.

Combination Therapy

In 1925, William H. Goeckerman at the Mayo Clinic proved the benefit of combining tar with UVB phototherapy to treat psoriasis. It clears psoriasis in more than 90% of patients and can produce long remissions. However, the use of this regimen has declined substantially, due to its messiness.

Other combination studies with UVB in adult populations have revealed mixed results: combination of UVB with topical corticosteroids has produced shortened remission time, and combination with calcipotriol has led to quicker and more complete clearing than with UVB therapy alone. For large plaque psoriasis in older children, the adult regimen of anthralin combined with measured graduated UVB exposure is efficacious and usually well tolerated. UVB may also be combined with systemic agents, such as MTX, acitretin, or the T-cell-targeted biologic agent alefacept, for more dramatic outcomes.

Photochemotherapy (PUVA)

PUVA is an acronym for psoralen combined with exposure to ultraviolet light A. PUVA therapy is not approved for children under 12 years of age, since the safety and efficacy of PUVA in children has not been established. Demonstrated risks include carcinogenicity, cataracts, actinic degeneration, and atypical pigmented lesions.

A number of researchers have suggested that combining PUVA with other treatment modalities, especially systemic retinoids (RePUVA), or rotating PUVA with other treatment forms (rotational therapy) may help in reducing the cumulative total dose.

Climatotherapy

Climatotherapy denotes the treatment for various types of diseases where a patient is relocated to areas around the world where the climate is more favorable for recovery. Climatotherapy may be particularly effective in the treatment of psoriasis. Climatotherapeutic areas around the world for psoriasis are: the Dead Sea (Israel), Red Sea (Egypt), Blue Lagoon in Grindavik (Iceland), Manitou Beach (Canada), Mavena Derma Center (Des Plaines, Ill., USA), and Soap Lake (Wash., USA). Although climatotherapy has been clinically demonstrated as viable, research in this area of medicine remains limited.

'Kangal hot spring with fish' or ichthyotherapy is yet another form of climatotherapy for psoriasis. Located in the central Anatolian region, the province of Sivas in Turkey is a thermal spring at an altitude of 1,405 m. The Kangal hot spring's water is 36°C with a pH of 7.3. The water is rich in minerals, including selenium, and harbors a great number of small fish from the Cyprinidae family, which suck at the scaly patches on the skin due to scarcity of natural food in the pool. It is the combination of balneotherapy, Kangal fish, and sun exposure that explains the success of this form of therapy, since the fish only remove the scale, and do not have any effect on the underlying inflammatory plaque. Due to this and reasons of animal welfare, keeping and use of Kangal fish for this purpose in private dermatologic practices seem inappropriate.

Systemic Therapy

As a general rule, systemic therapy for childhood psoriasis should only be used in extreme circumstances. The severity of the disease must be carefully assessed to determine whether the risk/benefit ration justifies a systemic treatment that has potential serious side effects for the child. Also, it should be kept in mind that children are likely to receive repeated treatments over their lifetime, exposing them to additional risk. Moreover, the long-term effects of some of the drugs are still unknown. Indications for systemic therapy for psoriasis in children are: resistant erythrodermic, pustular, or arthropathic psoriasis. Cyclosporin, MTX, and acitretin have all been used in children. Most experience with the use of these agents in children has been reported for cyclosporin in transplantation medicine, and for MTX in cancer chemotherapy. Because of lower tolerability of these agents in children and cumulative toxicities, treatment of psoriasis with the newer biologic agents, particularly the soluble tumor necrosis factor receptor fusion protein etanercept, is emerging.

Cyclosporin

Cyclosporin is an immunosuppressant drug widely used in post-allogeneic organ transplant to reduce the risk of organ rejection. Cyclosporin binds to the cytosolic protein cyclophilin (immunophilin) of T lymphocytes. This complex of cyclosporin and cyclophilin inhibits calcineurin, which is responsible for activating the transcription of IL-2. The inhibition of lymphokine production and interleukin release leads to a reduced function of effector T cells. Cyclosporin in doses of 2.5–5.0 mg/kg/day is approved for the treatment of adult patients with severe plaque psoriasis who have failed other treatment. Treatment duration is preferably limited to a period of 3 months to a maximum of 24 months. Cyclosporin has been used successfully and was well tolerated in cases of pediatric generalized pustular psoriasis [52], but pediatric use remains an off-label indication because there have not been adequate clinical trials in childhood psoriasis. Adverse effects of cyclosporine therapy include: hypertension, hyperlipidemia, nephropathy, headaches, tremors, hypertrichosis, and gingival hyperplasia. Baseline laboratory studies should include: serum creatinine, magnesium, potassium, lipids (fasting cholesterol and triglycerides), and complete blood count. Cyclosporin should be discontinued if reversibility of serum creatinine within 30% of the baseline cannot be attained after 2 dosage adjustments. Monitoring of blood pressure should occur every 2 weeks for the first 3 months of therapy, thereafter monthly if stable. Care should be taken to monitor patients who drink grapefruit juice or take other medications, which can interact with cyclosporin via cytochrome P-450.

Methotrexate

MTX is an antimetabolite initially developed and used in the treatment of cancer. It is used at lower doses as a treatment for inflammatory diseases, including psoriasis and psoriatic arthritis. In these cases, the inhibition of enzymes involved in purine metabolism is thought to be the main mode of action, leading to accumulation of adenosine, apoptosis and inhibition of T cells. MTX (administered either orally, or preferably subcutaneously) is approved for the treatment of psoriasis arthritis and severe adult psoriasis not responsive to other forms of therapy. A parallel use of low-dose MTX with TNF-α blockers, such as infliximab or etanercept, has been shown to markedly improve symptoms.

The safety and efficacy of MTX in the pediatric population has only been established for cancer chemotherapy and the treatment of polyarticular juvenile rheumatoid arthritis. When treating children with psoriasis, it may therefore be useful to keep in mind the recommendations for polyarticular juvenile rheumatoid arthritis. The lowest possible dose should be prescribed, preferably in the range 0.2–0.4 mg/kg per week [53]. Adverse effects of MTX therapy include: nausea and vomiting, teratogenicity, induction of abortion, acute bone marrow toxicity, and hepatotoxicity in the long term. Folic acid is given with MTX in order to lessen the associated gastrointestinal symptoms and anemia. All patients should undergo an initial assessment that includes: renal function tests, a complete blood count, liver function enzymes, and a pregnancy test (where applicable). These functions should be monitored during treatment. Because of its adverse effect profile on the liver, MTX should be avoided in children with liver disease, obesity, or diabetes (increased risk of cirrhosis). Abnormalities in a liver function test should prompt further investigation.

Acitretin

Acitretin is a second-generation retinoid, taken orally for the treatment of psoriasis and the congenital ichthyoses. It is a metabolite of etretinate, which was used prior to the introduction of acitretin, and discontinued because it had a narrow therapeutic index as well as a long elimination half-life. Acitretin is the least toxic systemic treatment for the treatment of severe resistant psoriasis. It binds to nuclear receptors that regulate gene transcription. They reduce epidermal hyperplasia and induce keratinocyte differentiation.

Acitretin is particularly useful in pustular and erythrodermic forms of psoriasis, even in the neonate [54]. Even though acitretin is not approved for pediatric use in psoriasis, most experience in the systemic treatment of childhood psoriasis has been reported with the retinoids, which therefore appear to be a second-line drug of choice. Nevertheless, there remains a concern that growth potential may be affected by the use of systemic retinoid therapy in children, especially in light of reports of premature epiphyseal closure. Ossification of interosseous ligaments and tendons on extremities and diffuse idiopathic skeletal hyperostosis have been reported with the chronic use of systemic retinoids in adults. The risk of this is minimized by using the lowest possible dose of acitretin (0.25–0.6 mg/kg), and discontinuing the drug when optimal result is achieved. Monitoring with a bone scan every 12–18 months has been recommended for children on systemic retinoids, but in contrast to the ichthyoses, continuous treatment over such periods of time are usually not necessary in psoriasis. Other side effects of concern are: pruritus, cheilitis, skin fragility, elevated serum lipids, elevation of liver enzymes, and pseudotumor cerebri. Again, baseline and follow-up monitoring are important when treating patients with this medication. Acitretin is a category X drug, contraindicated in pregnancy and lactation. Because acitretin can be metabolized into etretinate, which has a long half-life, females must avoid becoming pregnant for at least 2 years after discontinuing acitretin.

Therapy for psoriasis using oral retinoids and photochemotherapy (PUVA) for more dramatic effects, especially in generalized pustular and erythrodermic psoriasis, has been called RePUVA. The combination of oral retinoids with the newer biologic agents is currently under investigation.

Biologics

By definition, the term 'biologics' refers to a wide range of biologic products in medicine, such as vaccines, blood and blood components, allergenics, somatic cells, gene therapy, tissues, and recombinant therapeutic proteins, either isolated from natural sources – human, animal, or microorganism – or produced by biotechnology methods, usually recombinant DNA technology. Biologics are at the forefront of biomedical research, and are continuously being developed to treat a variety of medical conditions for which no other satisfactory treatments are available.

Advances in the understanding of the immunologic basis of psoriasis pathogenesis have led to targeted therapies in the form of biologics. These agents have gained popularity as allegedly safe, effective, and convenient alternatives for the treatment of chronic moderate-to-severe plaque psoriasis. Currently, 5 biologic agents are available for treatment of plaque psoriasis and/or psoriasis arthritis: the TNF-α antagonists (also effective in treatment of psoriasis arthritis) infliximab, etanercept, and adalimumab, and the T-cell-targeted biologics (only effective in treatment of skin psoriasis) alefacept and efalizumab; others are emerging, e.g. the IL-12/23 antagonist ustekinumab [for information on efalizumab, see chapter by Papp, pp. 95–106].

While only single case reports or small case series have so far been published with regard to the use of all other biologic agents, treatment of children and adolescents with plaque psoriasis with the soluble tumor necrosis factor receptor fusion protein etanercept has been assessed in a randomized double-blind placebo-controlled trial with 211 patients aged 4–17 years [55]: 57% of patients receiving 0.8 mg/kg etanercept achieved a 75% reduction in the PASI score from baseline (PASI 75), as compared to 11% of those receiving placebo. At week 36, after 24 weeks of open-label etanercept, rates of PASI 75 were 68 and 65% for patients initially assigned to etanercept or placebo, respectively. During the withdrawal period from week 36 to week 48, response was lost by 42% of patients assigned to placebo at a second randomization. With respect to pediatric arthritis patients, etanercept has been shown to successfully antagonize the persistent inflammatory stimulation attributed to TNF-α. Etanercept is approved for the treatment of juvenile rheumatoid arthritis at a dose of 0.8 mg/kg once weekly, and it has been proposed that controlling psoriasis arthritis early with etanercept may also be important in preventing disability.

Naturopathic Medicine

Naturopathic medicine (also known as 'natural medicine') is a complementary or alternative medicine which emphasizes the body's intrinsic ability to heal itself. Naturopaths prefer to use natural remedies, such as herbs and foods, rather than synthetic drugs. Naturopathic practice includes many different modalities. Practitioners emphasize a holistic approach to patient care, and base their practice upon the premise that nature will, given the right conditions, cure all maladies. Every individual has a healing force within himself that will heal all diseases, but this healing force requires certain conditions such as nutritious food, pure water, exercise, sunshine, fresh air, and rest (originally, the Hippocratic approach to healing diseases). Without these conditions, the body will be in a state of disease. Naturopathic medicine is practiced in many countries, but subject to different standards of regulation and levels of acceptance. The core set of interventions defined by the Council on Naturopathic Medical Education in North America includes: acupuncture and oriental medicine (traditional Chinese medicine, ayurveda), herbal medicine, homeopathy, nutrition, kinesiology, and reflexology. Naturopathy is viewed with much skepticism by some critics, including scientists and the medical profession, as it relies on unproven treatments, some of which are considered pseudoscience or quackery. Moreover, herbal medicine products (HMP) are not free of health hazards: 1 of 5 ayurvedic HMP produced in South Asia and available in Boston South Asian grocery stores was shown to contain potentially harmful levels of heavy metals (lead, mercury, and/or arsenic), and in our institute we have observed severe phototoxic skin reactions to ayurvedic HMP for treatment of skin conditions.

Conclusions

Management of psoriasis in children represents unique challenges. Treatment options are basically the same as for adults, but special care should be taken in order not to endanger the development or the future health of the child. Randomized controlled clinical trials involving children under the age of 12 years have only been reported for topical calcipotriol and corticosteroids. Phototherapy and conventional systemic therapy are of limited use because of lower tolerability and cumulative toxicities. For this reason, treatment with newer biologic agents is emerging. Finally, it is important to acknowledge a 'total care' package combining treatment, disease-specific education, and psychological support to cope with a possible lifelong skin condition.

References

1 Christophers E, Mrowietz U, Sterry W: Psoriasis, ed 2. Berlin, Blackwell, 2003.

2 Farber EM, Carlsen RA: Psoriasis in childhood. Calif Med 1966;105:415–420.

3 Beylot C, Puissant A, Bioulac P, et al: Particular clinical features of psoriasis in infants and children. Acta Derm Venereol Suppl (Stockh) 1979;87:95–97.

4 Morris A, Roger M, Fischer G, et al: Childhood psoriasis: a clinical review of 1,262 cases. Pediatr Dermatol 2001;18:188–198.

5 Swanbeck G, Inerot A, Mertinsson T, et al: Genetic counseling in psoriasis: empirical data on psoriasis among first-degree relatives of 3,095 psoriatic probands. Br J Dermatol 1997;137:939–942.

6 Nanda A, Kaur S, Kaur I, Kumar B: Childhood psoriasis: an epidemiological survey of 112 patients. Pediatr Dermatol 1990;7:19–21.

7 Dacou-Voutetakis C, Kakourou T: Psoriasis and blue sclerae in girls with Turner syndrome. J Am Acad Dermatol 1996;35:1002–1004.

8 Duffy DL, Spelman LS, Martin NG: Psoriasis in Australian twins. J Am Acad Dermatol 1993;29:428–434.

Yawalkar N (ed): Management of Psoriasis.
Curr Probl Dermatol. Basel, Karger, 2009, vol 38, pp 160–171

Management of Difficult to Treat Locations of Psoriasis

Scalp, Face, Flexures, Palm/Soles and Nails

Knud Kragballe

Department of Dermatology, Århus University Hospital, Århus, Denmark

Abstract

Psoriasis located on the scalp, face, skin folds, palms/soles and nails may require special consideration due to physical disability and discomfort, and because the treatment efficacy and safety may be different. There are many therapeutic approaches for psoriasis in difficult to treat locations. Only a few of the therapies have been evaluated for efficacy and safety in well-designed and well-controlled clinical studies. Furthermore, comparative studies are often lacking. This chapter describes management of psoriasis located on the scalp, face, skin folds, palm/soles and nails, with special focus on treatment with topical agents.

The choice of psoriasis therapy depends on the extent as well as the location of the disease. Body sites such as the scalp, face, skin folds, palms/soles and nails may require special consideration because they produce physical disability and discomfort, and because the drug efficacy and safety may be different. Furthermore, the clinical diagnosis of psoriasis may be difficult in certain locations, and sometimes psoriasis in special locations can only be recognized as a form of psoriasis by its association with more typical psoriasis elsewhere.

Psoriasis in special locations may occur along with psoriasis elsewhere on the body, or less frequently in isolation.

Management depends on the global assessment of disease severity. However, even psoriasis isolated to the scalp, face, palms, soles, genitalia or nails may impact the patients quality of life to a degree that systemic therapy, including biological therapy, may be indicated. According to the rule of tens, a score above 10 in the Psoriasis Area and Severity Index, greater than 10% of the body surface area involved, or a score above 10 in the Dermatology Life Quality Index indicates severe psoriasis [1]. Because Dermatology Life Quality Index scores may exceed 10 when the disease is present in difficult to treat locations, localized psoriasis may also be an indication for systemic therapy.

This chapter describes the management of difficult to treat locations of psoriasis with special focus on treatment with topical agents.

Scalp Psoriasis

Between 50 and 80% of patients with psoriasis report scalp psoriasis or concurrent psoriasis of the scalp and the body. In general, scalp psoriasis is difficult to treat due to the fact that the surface skin of the scalp is relatively inaccessible, reducing the effectiveness of topical therapies. Many therapeutic approaches for psoriasis exist, although only a few of the therapies currently used have been evaluated for efficacy in the setting of well-designed and well-controlled clinical studies of scalp psoriasis. Furthermore, head-to-head studies in comparison with established treatments for scalp psoriasis are lacking. Finally, patient satisfaction with currently available treatment is low, primarily due to the lack of efficacy and difficulty in applying the treatment, with convenience and a non-greasy formulation ranking high on patient's wishes for an ideal topical agent.

Topical preparations are the first-line treatments for scalp psoriasis, with the vehicle as well as the active ingredients being relevant to the efficacy and tolerability. The vehicles used can be either rinsed off as a shampoo or applied directly to the scalp (in a form of an alcohol-containing lotion, gel, foam, emulsion, cream, ointment or oil). Active ingredients include keratolytics, tar, dithranol, retinoids, antifungals, corticosteroids and vitamin D_3 analogues.

Corticosteroids

Topical corticosteroids are the mainstay of treatment for scalp psoriasis. Group III and IV corticosteroids produce fast and strong improvement [2]. They are also used for intermittent long-term therapy, despite the lack of data to support their safety and efficacy during prolonged use.

Corticosteroids delivered as an ointment are considered to be more potent than those delivered with other vehicles. Recent studies have, however, found that newer vehicles (such as lotions) can increase the ability of the active ingredients to penetrate the skin [3]. Also, clobetasol propionate and betamethasone valerate have become available in low-residue foam vehicles [4, 5] and in shampoo [6]. Delivered in such vehicles, the treatment becomes more convenient, which might improve patient compliance.

Vitamin D_3 Analogues

In clinical studies, tacalcitol formulations (cream, ointment or emulsion) have shown marked improvements without causing significant skin irritation [7]. Because the tacalcitol scalp emulsion is easy to wash out, it is well accepted by patients in markets where it is available.

Calcipotriol solution and cream is effective and safe for short-term as well as long-term treatment (52 weeks) [8]. For the short-term therapy, calcipotriol solution is almost as effective as betamethasone, although the corticosteroid has a stronger anti-pruritic effect [9]. Facial irritation has been reported with calcipotriol use for scalp psoriasis, although the effect seems to be transient and attenuates with continued use.

While the potent corticosteroids may be more effective for short-term use, the advantage of the vitamin D_3 analogues is that they are safe for prolonged use.

Combination of Corticosteroids and Vitamin D_3 Analogues

A new gel formulation of betamethasone dipropionate and calcipotriol has recently been developed for use in scalp psoriasis. The two-compound oily gel is more effective than either monotherapy [10]. Furthermore, it has been shown to be effective and safe for long-term (52 weeks) therapy without causing corticosteroid-related side effects [11]. This cosmetically acceptable combination of betamethasone dipropionate and calcipotriol was marketed in late 2008.

Tars

Coal tar preparations are still used for the treatment of scalp psoriasis. In an uncontrolled study, tar gel and shampoo was effective and produced a long-term remission in a significant number of patients [12]. However, coal tar has largely fallen out of favor due to its unpleasant smell and mutagenic potential.

Dithranol

Dithranol preparations may be effective. Their use is, however, limited by the staining and irritative capacity of dithranol. The treatment may be indicated for patients with resistant scalp psoriasis owing to its ability to produce a relatively long remission phase. Formulated in a new bio-wash-oil, dithranol has been shown to be effective and well tolerated in short-term therapy [13].

Keratolytics

In patients with thick scaling psoriasis, keratolytics (in particular salicylic acid) may be beneficial. Keratolytics may be used at the start of treatment to remove scaling, and thereby improve penetration of other topical therapies. Also, salicylic acid is used in fixed combinations with corticosteroids, such as betamethasone dipropionate. It has, however, not been demonstrated that salicylic acid increases the efficacy of the corticosteroid. Salicylic acid should not be mixed with vitamin D_3 analogues due to chemical incompatibility.

Any active ingredient is useless in very scaly scalp psoriasis. In these circumstances, petrolatum or a plant oil is applied at bedtime, sometimes occluded over night with a shower cap, and washed off in the morning. Salicylic acid and tar may be added to this pomade.

Other Topical Treatments

Topical and systemic anti-mycotics have been examined in scalp psoriasis. The results of these studies have been conflicting. Only when scalp psoriasis is present together with facial sebopsoriasis, does it seem justified to use antifungals. In these circumstances, ketoconazole can be used as shampoo.

Grenz ray therapy, which involve use of electrical magnetic radiation similar to X-rays but with reduced penetration, has been shown to be an effective and convenient alternative treatment for scalp psoriasis when topical agents have failed [14]. Because of the risk of skin carcinoma after repeated Grenz ray therapy, this therapy plays a limited role in the management of scalp psoriasis.

Summary

Scalp psoriasis is mainly treated with topicals. Corticosteroids and vitamin D_3 analogues are first-line agents. The combination of the rapid improvement from corticosteroids and the long-term steroid-sparing action of vitamin D_3 analogues may be the most suitable treatment for many patients. Pretreatment with keratolytics or oil may be necessary in thick scaling psoriasis. When topical treatment fails, systemic therapy with traditional or biological agents may be indicated.

Facial Psoriasis

Facial psoriasis is particularly common in children, and quality of life may be considerably impaired due to the visibility of the lesions. Three variants of facial psoriasis can be defined: hairline psoriasis, true facial psoriasis, and sebopsoriasis (fig. 1). While hairline psoriasis is regarded as part of scalp psoriasis, true facial psoriasis and sebopsoriasis are usually associated with severe long-standing psoriasis of early onset [15]. In facial psoriasis, photosensitivity should be considered. Corticosteroids,

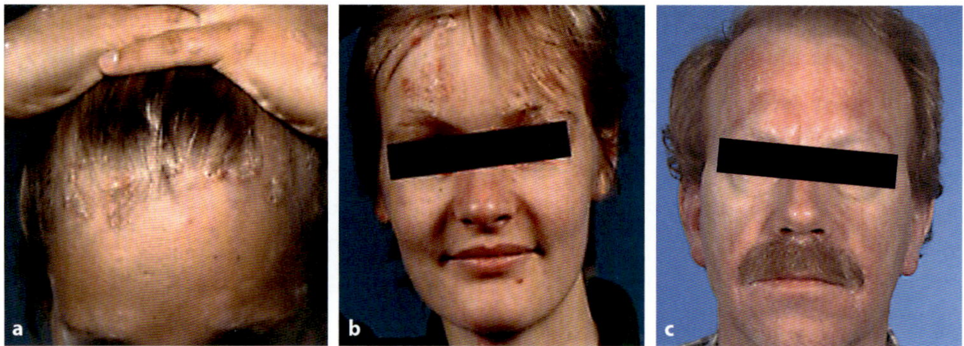

Fig. 1. Variants of facial psoriasis: hairline (**a**), facial plaques (**b**) and sebopsoriasis (**c**).

vitamin D_3 analogues and calcineurin inhibitors are the main topical treatments for facial psoriasis.

Corticosteroids

Topical corticosteroids have been used for many years as a first-choice treatment in facial psoriasis, despite the lack of double-blind randomized comparative studies. The side effects, such as skin atrophy, teleangiectasia and perioral dermatitis, have restricted the strength and duration of corticosteroid applications. In general, only low-strength topical corticosteroids (groups I and II) are recommended for facial psoriasis. A cream, applied once daily, is better accepted than ointment.

Vitamin D_3 Analogues

In case series, tacalcitol [16], calcitriol [17] and calcipotriol [18] have shown improvements in facial psoriasis. In an investigator-blinded comparative trial between calcitriol and calcipotriol, perilesional irritation was less severe following calcitriol compared to calcipotriol [19]. In contrast to topical corticosteroids, vitamin D_3 analogues are considered safe for long-term therapy.

Calcineurin Inhibitors

Tacrolimus ointment and pimecrolimus cream are labeled for treatment of atopic dermatitis. They are, however, also effective in facial psoriasis [20, 21]. Compared with the corticosteroid clobetasone butyrate (group II), tacrolimus 0.1% ointment has a similar efficacy and side effect profile over 6 weeks of treatment [22]. Due to their efficacy, together with minimal irritation, the calcineurin inhibitors are first-line treatments for facial psoriasis, particularly when long-term treatment is required.

Summary

See 'Summary, facial and flexural psoriasis'.

Psoriasis of Flexures

Flexural psoriasis, including genital and perianal psoriasis, is quite common and probably more frequent in elderly patients. In obese patients, flexural psoriasis may be accompanied by painful fissures and complicated by clinical signs of bacterial and mycotic infection.

Corticosteroids

Evidence for the efficacy of topical corticosteroids in flexural psoriasis is not available from double-blind randomized comparative trials. From clinical practice, low-strength topical corticosteroids (groups I and II) appear to be effective and safe for short-term treatment of flexural psoriasis. The risk of skin atrophy and striae restricts the use of potent corticosteroids. Recommendations are to use low-strength (group I and II) corticosteroid cream once daily for up to 4 weeks. If maintenance treatment is required, once-daily application for 2 consecutive days every week is considered safe.

Vitamin D_3 Analogues

Calcitriol cream and calcipotriol cream are effective and safe. In a comparative trial, calcitriol was superior to calcipotriol [19]. Furthermore, skin irritation was more common with calcipotriol. In conclusion, vitamin D_3 analogues (in particular calcitriol) are effective and safe in flexural psoriasis. In contrast to corticosteroids, vitamin D_3 analogues can be used for long-term therapy.

Calcineurin Inhibitors

Although not labeled for psoriasis, tacrolimus ointment [20], as well as pimecrolimus cream [23], has been shown to be efficacious and safe for the treatment of

Efalizumab has been studied in palmoplantar psoriasis resistant to traditional systemic treatment. In a randomized, placebo-controlled trial of palmoplantar plaque psoriasis, 46% of the 52 efalizumab-treated patients obtained a satisfactory improvement after 3 months [35]. In a case series of palmoplantar psoriasis, efalizumab produced excellent improvements in both the plaque (n = 11) and pustular-type (n = 6) forms [36; for information on efalizumab, see chapter by Papp, pp. 95–106].

Summary

Topical therapies have modest efficacy in palmoplantar psoriasis. In moderate to severe cases, traditional systemic therapy including PUVA is indicated. For recalcitrant cases, biological agents are recommended. It remains to be determined which systemic therapy has the most favorable efficacy-to-safety ratio in palmoplantar psoriasis.

Nail Psoriasis

Nails are affected in about 10–50% of patients. The incidence of nail psoriasis is considered to be higher in the presence of psoriatic arthritis. Often nail psoriasis is associated with severe disease. Psoriatic nail disease causes significant psychological stress and may impair patients in social settings and in the workplace [37].

There are only few and small controlled clinical studies related to existing topical systemic and biological therapies. Therefore, no consistent treatment approach has been advocated for nail psoriasis. The choice of treatment for nail psoriasis depends on the clinical features of the disease and specific patient factors. If the nail changes are mild, treatment may not be indicated. If nail psoriasis is the sole manifestation of the skin disease and arthritis is absent, topical therapy is an appropriate initial approach. Systemic therapy is often required if patients fail to respond to topical therapy, if significant skin or joint disease is present, or if their nail disease is especially severe (i.e. pustular nail disease).

Topical Therapy

Topical therapies include corticosteroid and calcipotriol therapy. Onycholysis may benefit if the nail is clipped back to the point of the nail plate attachment, and the nail bed treated topically. In cases of severe nail dystrophy, topical treatment may be proceeded by chemical removal of the nail plate with 40% urea ointment under occlusion. Potent corticosteroids may be used without occlusion, rubbed into the nail fold [38, 39]. Alternatively, corticosteroids may be injected into the nail fold or the nail bed [40]. With a needleless device, this can be done without local anesthesia [41]. Calcipotriol cream can be useful when there is subungual hyperkeratosis and nail thickening [39]. Calcipotriol has the advantage of avoiding the risk of atrophy with long-term use. Also, it may be beneficial to use a combination of a topical steroid and calcipotriol [42].

Systemic Therapy

Improvement in psoriatic skin disease during systemic therapy is often accompanied by improved nail changes. Oral acitretin makes the nail plate thin. This reduces subungual hyperkeratosis. On the other hand, pitting and onycholysis may be exacerbated. Pustulation is often improved by acitretin [38, 43]. Methotrexate and cyclosporin improve nail psoriasis to some degree, but are not usually recommended for nail psoriasis alone. Acrodermatitis continua of Hallopeau is an exception [43, 44].

Biological therapy for psoriasis and psoriatic arthritis may benefit psoriatic nail disease. In a 1-year study with infliximab, there was a marked and sustained nail improvement [45]. It was noted that the improvement was most rapid and most complete for red spots in the lunula and for splinter hemorrhages, while pitting was the slowest to respond. More studies on the impact of biological therapy on nail psoriasis are forthcoming, and will likely increase our ability to improve treatment of this important manifestation of psoriasis.

Summary

The effect of topical agents is usually disappointing in nail psoriasis. Also, traditional systemic therapy can be less effective for nail psoriasis than for psoriasis elsewhere. In severe nail psoriasis, biological therapy may become the treatment of choice.

References

1 Finlay AY: Current severe psoriasis and the rule of tens. Br J Dermatol 2005;152:861–867.

2 Pauporte M, Maibach H, Lowe N, et al: Fluocinolone acetonide topical oil for scalp psoriasis. J Dermatol Treat 2004;15:360–364.

3 Stein L: Clinical studies of a new vehicle formulation for topical corticosteroids in the treatment of psoriasis: J Am Acad Dermatol 2005;53(suppl 1): S39–S49.

4 Gottlieb AB, Ford RO, Spellman MC: The efficacy and tolerability of clobetasol propionate foam 0.05% in the treatment of mild to moderate plaque-type psoriasis of nonscalp regions. J Cutan Med Surg 2003;7:185–192.

5 Andreassi L, Giannetti A, Milani M, Scalp Investigators Group: Efficacy of betamethasone valerate mousse in comparison with standard therapies on scalp psoriasis: an open, multicentre, randomized, controlled, cross-over study on 241 patients: Br J Dermatol 2003;148:134–138.

6 Jarratt M, Breneman D, Gottlieb AB, Poulin Y, Liu Y, Foley V: Clobetasol propionate shampoo 0.05%: a new option to treat patients with moderate to severe scalp psoriasis. J Drugs Dermatol 2004;3:367–373.
7 Ruzicka T, Trompke C: Treatment of scalp psoriasis: an effective and safe tacalcitol emulsion. Hautarzt 2004;55:165–170.
8 Barnes L, Altmeyer P, Forstrom L, Stenstrom MH: Long-term treatment of psoriasis with calcipotriol scalp solution and cream. Eur J Dermatol 2000;10: 199–204.
9 Duweb GA, Abuzariba O, Rahim M, al-Taweel M, Abdullah SA: Scalp psoriasis: topical calcipotriol 50 micrograms/g/ml solution vs. betamethasone valerate 1% lotion. Int J clin Pharmacol Res 2000;20:483–487.
10 Jemec GBE, Ganslandt C, Ortonne JP, Poulin Y, Burden AD, de Unamuno, Berne B, Figueiredo A, Anstad J: A new scalp formulation of calcipotriene plus betamethasone compared with its active ingredients and the vehicle in the treatment of scalp psoriasis: a randomized, double-blind controlled trial. J Am Acad Dermatol 2008;59:455–463.
11 Luger T, Kidson P, Cambazard F, Larsen FG: A 1-year randomized, double-blind safety study of long-term treatment of a new gel formulation containing calcipotriene plus betamethasone dipropionate in scalp psoriasis. J Am Acad Dermatol 2008; 58 (suppl 2):AB134.
12 Langer A, Wolska H, Hebborn P: Treatment of psoriasis of the scalp with coal tar gel and shampoo preparations. Cutis 1983;32:295–296.
13 Wulff-Woesten A, Ohlendorf D, Henz BM, Hass N: Dithranol in an emulsifying oil base (bio-wash-oil) for the treatment of psoriasis of the scalp. Skin Pharmacol 2004;17:91–97.
14 Lindelof B: Grenz ray therapy in dermatology: an experimental, clinical and epidemiological study. Acta Derm Venereol Suppl (Stockh) 1987;132:1–67.
15 Park JY, Kim JH, Choe YB: Facial psoriasis: Comparison of patients with and without facial involvement. J Am Dermatol 2004;50:582–584.
16 Tadaki T, Kato T, Tagami H: Topical active vitamin D-3 analogue, 1,24-dihydroxycholecalciferol, an effective new treatment for facial seborrhoeic dermatitis. J Dermatolog Treat 1996;7:139–140.
17 Langer A, Stapor V, Verjans H, Elzerman J: Calcitriol ointment in the treatment of facial, hairline and retroauricular chronic plaque psoriasis. J Dermatolog Treat 1996;7:(suppl I):S15–S18.
18 Kienbaum S, Lehmann P, Ruzicka T: Topical calcipotriol in the treatment of flexural psoriasis. Br J Dermatol 1996;135:647–650.
19 Ortonne JP, Humbert P, Nicolas JF, Tsankov N, Tonev SD, Janin A, et al: Intraindividual comparison of the cutaneous safety and efficacy of calcitriol 3 mcg g^{-1} ointment and calcipotriol 50 mcg g^{-1} ointment on chronic plaque psoriasis localized in facial, hairline, retroauriculair or flexural areas. Br J Dermatol 2003;148:326–333.
20 Lebwohl M, Freeman A, Chapman MS, Feldman SR, Hartle JE, Henning A: Tacrolimus ointment is effective for facial and intertriginous psoriasis. J Am Acad Dermatol 2004;51:723–730.
21 Jacobi A, Braetigam, Mahler V, Schultz E, Herti M: Pimecrolimus 1% cream in the treatment of facial psoriasis: a 16-week open-label study. Dermatology 2008;216:133–136.
22 Kleyn CE, Woodcock D, Sharpe GR: The efficacy of 0.1% tacrolimus ointment compared with clobetasonebutyrate 0.05% ointment in patients with facial flexural or genital psoriasis (abstract). Br J Dermatol 2005;153(suppl 1):33.
23 Gribetz C, Ling M, Lebwohl M, Pariser D, Draelos Z, Gottlieb AB, Zaias N, Chen DM, Parneix-Spake A, Hultsch T, Menter A: Picmecrolimus cream 1% in the treatment of intertriginous psoriasis: a double-blind, randomized study. J Am Acad Dermatol 2004;51:731–738.
24 Kreuter A, Sommer A, Hyun J, Brautigam M, Brockmeyer NH, Altmeyer P, Gambichler T: 1% pimecrolimus, 0.005% calcipotriol, and 0.1% betamethasone in the treatment of intertriginous psoriasis: a double-blind, randomized controlled study. Arch Dermatol 2006;142:1138–1143.
25 Griffiths CEM, Christophers E, Barker JNWN, Chalmers RJG, Chimenti S, Krueger GG, Leonardi C, Menter A, Ortonne J-P, Fry L: A classification of psoriasis vulgaris according phenotype. Br J Dermatol 2007;156:258–262.
26 Pettey AA, Balkrishnan R, Rapp SR, Fleischer AB, Feldman S: Patients with palmo-plantar psoriasis have more physical disability and discomfort than patients with other forms of psoriasis: implications for clinical practice. J Am Acad Dermatol 2003;49: 271–275.
27 Yiannias JA, Winkelmann RK, Connolly SM: Contact sensitivities in palmo-plantar pustulosis. Contact Dermatitis 1998;39:108–111.
28 Kragballe K, Larsen FG: A hydrocolloid occlusive dressing plus triamcinolone acetonide cream is superior to clobetasol cream in palmo-plantar pustulosis. Acta Derm Venereol 1991;71:540–542.
29 Duweb GA, Abuzariba O, Rahim M, al-Taweel M, al-Alem S, Abdulla SA: Occlusive versus nonocclusive calcipotriol ointment treatment for palmoplantar psoriasis. Int J Tissue React 2001;23:59–62.

30 Lassus A, Greiger JM: Acitretin and etretinate in the treatment of palmoplantar pustulosis: a double-blind comparative trial. Br J Dermatol 1988;119:755–759.

31 Jansen CT, Malmiharju T: Inefficacy of topical methoxalen plus UVA for palmoplantar pustulosis. Acta Derm Venereol 1981;61:354–356.

32 De Rie MA, Van Eendenburg JP, Versnick AC, Stolk LM, Bos JD, Westerhof W: A new psoralen-containing gel for topical PUVA therapy: development, and treatment results in patients with palmoplantar and plaque-type psoriasis, and hyperkeratotic eczema. Br J Dermatol 1995;132:964–969.

33 Aubin F, Vigan M, Puzenat E, et al: Evaluation of a novel 308-nm monochromatic excimer light delivery system in dermatology: a pilot study in different chronic localized dermatoses. Br J Dermatol 2005; 152:99–103.

34 Erkko P, Granlund H, Remitz A, et al: Double-blind placebo-controlled study of long-term low-dose cyclosporin in the treatment of palmoplantar pustulosis. Br J Dermatol 1998;139:997–1004.

35 Leonardi C, Sofen H, Krell J, Caro I, Compton P, Sobell JM: Phase IV study to evaluate the safety and efficacy of efalizumab for treatment of hand and foot plaques psoriasis. J Am Acad Dermatol 2007; 56(suppl 2), AB84, poster 532.

36 Fretzin S, Crowley J, Jones L, Young M, Sobell J: Successful treatment of hand and foot psoriasis with efalizumab therapy. J Drugs Dermatol 2006;5:838–846.

37 de Jong EM, Seegers BA, Gulinck MK, Boezemann JB, van de Kerkhof PC: Psoriasis of the nails is associated with disability in a large number of patients: results of a recent interview with 1,728 patients. Dermatology 1996;193:300–303.

38 Piraccini BM, Trosti A, Iorizzo M, Misciali C: Pustular psoriasis of the nails: treatment and long-term follow-up of 46 patients. Br J Dermatol 2001; 144:1000–1005.

39 Tosti A, Piraccini BM, Cameli N, et al: Calcipotriol ointment in nail psoriasis: a controlled double-blind comparison with betamethasone dipropionate and salicylic acid. Br J Dermatol 1998;139:655–659.

40 de Berker DA, Lawrence CM: A simplified protocol of steroid injection for psoriatic nail dystrophy. Br J Dermatol 1998;138:90–95.

41 Bleeker JJ: Intralesional triamcinolone acetonide using the Port-O-Jet and needle injections in localized dermatoses. Br J Dermatol 1997;91:97–101.

42 Rigopoulos D, Ioannides D, Prastitis N, Katsambas A: Nail psoriasis: a combined treatment using calcipotriol cream and clobetasol propionate cream (letter). Acta Derm Venereol 2002;82:140.

43 Mahrle G, Schulze HJ, Farber L, Weidinger G, Steigleder GK: Low-dose short-term cyclosporine versus etretinate in psoriasis: improvement of skin, nail and joint involvement. J Am Acad Dermatol 1995;32:78–88.

44 Feliciani C, Zampetti A, Forleo P, et al: Nail psoriasis: combined therapy with systemic cyclosporine and topical calcipotriol. J Cutan Med Surg 2004;8: 122–125.

45 Rich P, Griffiths CEM, Reich K, Nestle F, Scher RK, Li S, Xu S, Hsu M-C, Guzzo C: Baseline nail disease in patients with moderate to severe psoriasis and response to treatment with infliximab during 1 year. J Am Acad Dermatol 2008;58:224–231.

Prof. Knud Kragballe, MD
Department of Dermatology, Århus University Hospital, Århus Sygehus
P.P.Ørums Gade 11
DK–8000 Århus C (Denmark)
Tel. +45 8949 1856, Fax +45 8949 1850, E-Mail knudkrag@rm.dk

Yawalkar N (ed): Management of Psoriasis.
Curr Probl Dermatol. Basel, Karger, 2009, vol 38, pp 172–189

Future Perspectives in the Treatment of Psoriasis

K. Wippel-Slupetzky · G. Stingl

Department of Dermatology, Division of Immunology, Allergy and Infectious Diseases, Medical University of Vienna, Vienna, Austria

Abstract

All available antipsoriatic therapies are of symptomatic character. Treatments established so far are limited in their use due to side effects or lack of efficacy resulting in poor quality of life for affected people. Development of new therapeutic approaches would not only broaden our armamentarium against psoriasis, but could also increase our understanding of the pathogenesis of this disease. In brief, 2 main targets represent attractive candidates, either the keratinocyte itself or the immune system. Promising therapeutic strategies include: (1) the search for new psoriasis susceptibility genes and their resulting phenotypes; (2) the interference with certain parts of cell signaling pathways that are involved in inflammatory processes; (3) the inhibition or elimination of activated T lymphocytes, e.g. by blocking of costimulatory signals or by deviation of a pathogenic immune response into a nonpathogenic one; (4) the blockade of proinflammatory cytokines; (5) the inhibition of leukocyte extravasation or trafficking; (6) the inhibition of angiogenesis. Some of these strategies are in phase 2 trials, others have already reached phase 3 status and are close to being approved by medicine agencies, and some are still visions of the future. This book chapter will give an overview of these new treatment strategies.

Psoriasis is a common chronic inflammatory skin disorder that affects about 2–3% of the world's population. Depending on the degree of severity and activity of the disease, several topical, physical and systemic therapies are available nowadays.

They either target selective immune mechanisms involved in the disease process or are of auxiliary value. Up to now, all currently available therapies are only symptomatic. For localized and mild forms, topical corticosteroids, vitamin D_3 analogs (calcipotriene), retinoids (tazarotene), tars, anthralin and phototherapy are good therapeutic options. Conventional systemic therapies for severe psoriasis include oral retinoids, methotrexate, cyclosporine and PUVA. These established treatments are often sufficient for disease control, but all of them have their limitations. After long-term use 'escape mechanisms' may occur, resulting in loss of response. Alternatively, a high potential for considerable adverse effects impairing quality of life may force treating physicians to terminate otherwise effective therapies. In the last years, an increased understanding of the pathophysiology of psoriasis has enabled the development of new targeted biological agents. Although these biologics have ushered in a new therapeutic era by revolutionizing the management of severe psoriasis, our long-term experience with these compounds is still limited, both with regard to efficacy and, more importantly, safety. Additionally, loss of efficacy as well as disease unresponsiveness have also been observed for biologics. For that reason, there is a need for new highly effective and safe therapy options for both topical and systemic use. If one takes the complex pathogenesis of psoriasis into consideration, there are diverse targets for therapeutic interventions. This book chapter aims at summarizing new treatment approaches for psoriasis (table 1).

The pathogenesis of this highly inflammatory disease has long been a matter of debate. Controversy exists as to whether psoriasis starts as a primary abnormality in keratinocytes or is the consequence of an altered immune response against an as yet undefined antigen. The first hypothesis claims that 1 or more genetically determined molecular lesions in indigenous cells of the skin (e.g. keratinocytes) induce an altered activation of these cells. In fact, aberrant signaling and transcription factor activation can serve as a reasonable explanation for the defective growth control and differentiation of psoriatic keratinocytes [1], as well as for the occurrence of an inflammatory tissue response being induced by cytokines produced by activated keratinocytes such as IL-1, IL-6, IL-8, IFN-γ, TNF-α, TGF-α and granulocyte/macrophage colony-stimulating factor [2]. This could result in an antigen-independent activation, adhesion and attraction of T lymphocytes. Zenz et al. [3] developed a mouse model, in which the elimination of the central transcription factor JunB in epidermal keratinocytes leads to a phenotype that greatly resembles psoriasis including arthritis. There was not only a disturbed epidermal differentiation, but also dermal changes including inflammation and expression of chemokines/cytokines recruiting neutrophils and macrophages. From a conceptual viewpoint, it is certainly remarkable that epidermal alterations are sufficient to initiate both skin lesions and arthritis in psoriasis. JunB is a gene localized in PSORS6, 1 of the at least 20 psoriasis susceptibility regions that have been identified so far.

According to the second hypothesis, psoriasis is the result of an abnormal immune response to an as yet undefined autoantigen or microbial antigens, e.g. streptococcal, with molecular homology to certain self proteins [4]. It is not yet clear where the psoriatic immune response begins. Lymphoid tissues such as tonsils are certainly a good candidate as identical TCR patterns have been described in tonsillar T cells after streptococcal infection and skin-homing T cells in peripheral blood and skin. On the other hand, nonlesional psoriatic skin contains a small reservoir of pathogenic T cells that can be expanded by stimuli derived from certain types of cutaneous dendritic cells [5]. In any event, one can assume that T cells attracted to and/or expanded in the skin do not only cause inflammation, but also, through keratinocyte activation,

Table 1. New systemic therapeutic perspectives in the treatment of psoriasis

Strategies	Areas of interest
Inhibition of growth factors	tyrosine kinase inhibitors
P38 MAPK inhibitors	BMS-582949
JAK/STAT pathway inhibitors	JAK3 antibody (CP-690,550)
PDE-4 inhibitors	apremilast (CC-10004)
Protein kinase C inhibitor	AEB071
Inhibition of T cell activation/elimination of activated T cells	CD3 antibody (Hum29) CD4 antibody (OKT4a) IL-2-diphteria toxin fusion protein (DAB398IL-2, Ontak®) calcineurin inhibitors (ISA 247, Voclosporin®)
Blockade of costimulatory signals	CTLA-4 Ig (abatacept, Orencia®, BMS-188667) CD80 antibody (IDEC-114, galiximab)
Deviation of Th1 and Th17 to Th2 responses	IL-4 IL-10 (Tenovil™) IL-12/23 p40 antibodies (CNTO 1275, ustekinumab, Stelara™, ABT-874)
Inhibition of proinflammatory cytokines	TNF-α (golimumab) INF-γ (fontolizumab, HuZAF®) INF-α (MEDI-545) IL-6 antibody (tocilizumab, Actemra®) IL-8 antibody (HuMab 10F8) IL-18/IL-1 release inhibitor P2x7 (CE-224,535)
Blocking of leukocyte extravasation/ trafficking	Pan-selectin antagonist (bimosiamose, TBC1269, efomycine)
Antiangiogenesis	VEGF antagonist (AE-941, Neovastat®)

enhanced production of growth factors resulting in acanthosis, parakeratosis and neoangiogenesis.

Interference with Upregulated Signal Transduction Pathways in Psoriatic Skin

In normal skin, keratins 5/14 are found in the basal layer, whereas in psoriatic skin they reach the spinous layer [6]. In contrast, keratins 10/1, which are normally expressed in suprabasal keratinocytes, are considerably reduced. Keratins 6/16, which usually play an essential role in wound healing, are both strongly expressed in psoriatic epidermis. Classic therapies such as dithranol, tar, vitamin D derivates, retinoids and methotrexate are said to inhibit keratinocyte hyperproliferation, beside other effects. All these therapies have their limitations, either concerning their efficacy, applicability, side effects and resulting quality of life issues. Therefore, we are seeking innovative strategies.

Due to an increased understanding of signaling pathways that are operative in cell cycle regulation and gene transcription [7], new potential targets in keratinocytes and/or inflammatory cells could be identified.

Inhibition of Growth Factors (e.g. Epidermal Growth Factor) and Subsequent Activation of Receptor Tyrosine Kinases

The epidermal growth factor receptor and its ligands represents one of the main switches regulating central biological processes such as cell division, cell death, differentiation and tumorigenesis [for a review, see 8]. Overexpression of multiple EGRF ligands is also a hallmark of the psoriatic epidermis. To date, there exist individual case reports of clinical improvement of psoriasis with tyrosine kinase inhibitors (e.g. imatinib) that were given primarily against various types of cancer [9]. However, prospective, randomized studies are still missing.

p38 MAPK Inhibitors

Certain signals from the cell surface are transduced into changes in cell cycle kinetics and/or gene expression via intracellular protein cascades such as MAPK [10]. Four classical MAPK have been described [11]: the extracellular signal-regulated kinases 1 and 2 (ERK 1/2), the p38 MAPK, the c-jun amino-terminal kinases and atypical MAPK (ERK 3 and ERK 5). P38 MAPK cascades are involved in the production of TNF by macrophages in response to stimulation with lipopolysaccharides [12] and are activated in many cell types, also keratinocytes, in response to TNF signaling. Johansen et al. [13] showed that both ERK 1/2 and p38 activity are increased in psoriatic skin, indicating a possible role in the development of the disease.

Several p38 inhibitors have been tested in clinical trials that were discontinued because of considerable side effects such as CNS and liver toxicity [14]. New p38 MAPK inhibitors that are unable to cross the brain-blood barrier are now being tested in clinical trials. As an example, the study using the compound BMS-582949 (Bristol-Myers-Squibb) is currently recruiting participants for a placebo-controlled phase II study. There are 4 treatment groups, either receiving tablets containing 10, 30, 100 mg BMS-582949 or placebo. The estimated study completion is December 2009.

JAK/STAT Pathway Inhibitors

JAK are a small family of protein tyrosine kinases that are linked to cytokine receptors and consist of JAK1, JAK2, JAK3 and the tyrosine kinase-2. JAKS are activated by the hematopoietic cytokine family and by interferons that target the STAT family of transcription factors. Unlike other JAKS, which are widely expressed and bind several cytokine receptors, JAK3 is an attractive candidate for drug development since it has limited tissue distribution and is activated by IL-2, IL-4, IL-7, IL-9, IL-15 and IL-21 [15]. The first orally available selective JAK3 antibody (CP-690, 550) effectively prevented transplant rejection in animal models and inhibited delayed hypersensitivity. Its role in treating autoimmune diseases has yet to be evaluated.

STAT are a family of latent cytoplasmatic proteins involved in transmitting extracellular signals to the nucleus. Among the STAT, targeting STAT 3 may be of particular therapeutic benefit. STAT3 is involved in the regulation of cell migration, survival and proliferation, and is activated in psoriasis. Sano et al. [16] described a transgenic mouse model with keratinocytes expressing constitutively active STAT3. These mice develop a phenotype resembling psoriasis after wounding or even spontaneously. The onset of psoriatic lesions could be inhibited by abrogation of the STAT3 function, and established lesions could be reversed.

Phosphodiesterase 4 Inhibitors

The phosphodiesterases (PDE) are enzymes which specifically degrade the phosphodiester bond in the second messenger molecules cAMP and cGMP. So far, 11 different PDE have been described. Among them, PDE4 is the major cAMP-metabolizing enzyme found in many inflammatory cells such as T cells, macrophages, neutrophils and eosinophils, but is also expressed in keratinocytes and fibroblasts. Since the late 1980s, PDE4 inhibitors have been under investigation as anti-inflammatory therapies against asthma and chronic obstructive pulmonary disease. So far, none of the agents developed have reached the market, mainly due to a lack of efficacy caused by the narrow therapeutic window of these inhibitors. Dose-limiting side effects like nausea, diarrhea, vomiting and abdominal pain are the main obstacle. Due to the broad anti-inflammatory activity of PDE4 inhibitors, their possible use in the treatment of atopic dermatitis and psoriasis was examined. Some of them showed strong anti-inflammatory action in models of allergic and irritant skin affections. Recently presented results from a randomized 260-patient multicenter study demonstrated that 24.4% of patients treated with 20 mg b.i.d. of oral apremilast (CC-10004) had a PASI 75 after 84 days, compared to 10.3% in the placebo arm [presented at the 66th Ann Meet Am Acad Dermatol, Feb 2008]. Based on these promising results, the dosage will be raised to 30 mg b.i.d. and the duration of dosing will be expanded up to 6 months.

Protein Kinase C Inhibitors

AEB071 is an attractive tool, which is an inhibitor of protein kinase C (PKC) and consequently blocks early T cell activation as measured by IL-2 production and also keratinocytes. It strongly and selectively inhibits the classical (α, β) and the novel θ-PKC isoforms, with lesser activity for the δ-, ε- and η-PKC isoforms. These PKC isoforms play an important role in signaling pathways downstream of the T cell receptor and the CD28 receptor. Originally developed for the prevention of acute rejection of solid organ allotransplantations, recent studies demonstrated good efficacy in the treatment of psoriasis. In a recently published study, AEB071 was administered orally to 32 patients with severe plaque psoriasis for 2 weeks. There were 4 cohorts of 8 patients each, who received AEB071 in a dose-escalating fashion (ranging from 25 to 300 mg b.i.d.); 2 patients per group received placebo. There was a dose-dependent improvement, showing a PASI 75 for 69% of the treatment group receiving 300 mg b.i.d. [17]. Larger patient cohorts and longer treatment periods will provide further information about the potential of AEB071 as a psoriasis therapy.

Selective Modulation/Inhibition of the Immune/Inflammatory Response

The most commonly used immunosuppressive drugs like cyclosporine and corticosteroids are directed against a myriad of targets involved in the pathogenesis of psoriasis, resulting in a high efficiency but with several adverse effects. Generating more selective therapies might have advantages over classic therapies.

Inhibition of T Cell Activation/Elimination of Activated T Cells

The first hints that T cells are critically involved in the pathogenesis of psoriasis occurred in the mid-1980s, when cyclosporine dramatically cleared psoriatic plaques in clinical trials [18]. Calcineurin inhibitors such as cyclosporine downregulate gene expression in type-1 T cells, Th17 cells and TIP-DC (TNF- and inducible nitric oxide synthase-producing dendritic cells) [19] and show very good efficacy, but side effects (nephrotoxicity, elevation of blood pressure) restrict their long term use. ISA 247 (Voclosporin; Isotechinka, Edmonton, Alta. Canada) has a modification of the functional group at the amino acid 1 residue, and is said to be less nephrotoxic. In a placebo-controlled 4-arm phase III study, 47% of the group receiving the highest dose (0.4 mg/kg b.i.d.) reached a PASI 75 score after 12 weeks, as compared to 4% of the placebo group; 7 out of 113 patients in this group showed mild-to-moderate glomerular filtration rate reductions. Response and side effects were dose-dependent. In comparison to cyclosporine, it seems to have a better outcome concerning changes in renal function [20]. In the early 1990s, there were the first trials testing T-cell-specific antibodies. Small studies with Hum29, an anti-CD3 antibody (directed against all T cells) [21], and OKT4a, an anti-CD4 antibody (directed against T helper cells), were conducted and demonstrated efficacy [22], but larger clinical trials are missing.

The hypothesis that activated T cells are important for disease maintenance was supported when denileukin diftitox, which is a fusion protein of IL-2 and diphtheria toxin protein fragments, was used in clinical trails. Named Ontak® (DAB398IL-2), the fusion protein showed good efficacy in about 40% of patients with severe psoriasis, but its use is limited by its toxicity [23]. The reason why certain patients did not improve or even deteriorated was probably due to the fact that Ontak eliminates not only activated T cells, but also CD25+ T regulatory cells.

T cell-activation requires the delivery of 3 signals. First, the antigen that is bound to class I or II major histocompatibility complex antigens on the surface of an antigen-presenting cell (APC) interacts with the T cell receptor and determines the specificity of the response. Second, the display of costimulatory molecules is critical for the strength of the immunological synapse and, thus, for the magnitude of the response. Third, it is the elaboration of immunomodulatory cytokines that determines the quality of the response.

Blockade of Costimulatory Molecules

Potential targets for interventional therapies are: (1) the leukocyte function-associated antigen 1 (LFA-1) and the intercellular adhesion molecule 1 (ICAM-1), inhibited by the monoclonal antibody efalizumab; (2) CD2 and LFA-3, targeted by the LFA-3-IgG1 fusion protein alefacept; (3) CD80/CD86 and CD28/CD152 = cytotoxic T-lymphocyte antigen 4 (CTLA4), blocked by CTLA4Ig (abatacept, Orencia™, BMS-188667) and the CD80-antibody IDEC-114. CD80 and CD86, which are mainly expressed on activated APC and on a subset of activated T cells, interact with CD28 and deliver a costimulatory signal that leads to T cell activation. As a regulatory factor, CTLA4 is consecutively upregulated on the T cell surface, resulting in T cell deactivation and downregulation of the immune response [24]. CTLA4Ig, a soluble fusion protein of the extracellular domain of human CD152 and a fragment of the Fc portion of human IgG1, binds to CD80 and CD86 on APC, and therefore inhibits the CD28-mediated costimulatory signal for T cell activation. In an open-label phase-I study including 43 patients with stable plaque psoriasis, CTLA4Ig (abatacept) was administered intravenously on days 1, 3, 16 and 29 at doses between 0.5 and 50 mg/kg. Results obtained showed that CTLA4-Ig has a moderate, dose-dependent antipsoriatic effect; 1/5 patients in the 1-mg/kg group achieved a 50% or greater improvement in their Physician's Global Assessment (PGA) of disease activity, as did 5/6 patients in the 25-mg/kg group and 4/5 patients in the 50-mg/kg group. This was accompanied by histological changes, such as normalization of keratinocyte differentiation and proliferation and a decrease in CD3+ T cells, mostly at the dermal-epidermal junction [25].

IDEC-114 (galiximab), a monoclonal antibody that specifically binds CD80, inhibits the interaction between CD80 and CD28 without influencing the T-cell-regulatory interaction of CD80 and CTLA4 (CD152). In an open-label dose-finding study, 24 psoriasis patients received 1 infusion of IDEC-114 in 6 different doses ranging from 0.05 up to 15 mg/kg [26]. Only patients in the 10-mg/kg group showed a PASI 25 improvement on day 29 of the study. The other treatment groups had no significant changes in their PGA assessments.

Immunodeviation

One can safely assume that Th1 and Th17 cells, as well as the cytokines secreted by them and acting upon them, are critical players in the pathogenesis of psoriasis. Similar to what has been accomplished in autoimmune diseases in experimental animals, attempts have been made to switch a pathogenic situation into a nonpathogenic one [27].

Interleukin 4

IL-4 was first described in 1986 and is, together with IL-13, the leading cytokine operative in the Th2 pathway. In a prospective open-label dose-escalation study, 22 patients received IL-4 subcutaneously over a period of 6 weeks. IL-4 was administered 3 times daily for 5 days a week in different dosages (0.05, 0.1, 0.2, 0.3 or 0.5 μg/kg). After 3 weeks, the dosage was elevated to the next level. The treatment was well tolerated, only in the highest dosage-group were side effects (such as headache and influenza-like symptoms) observed. Eighteen patients demonstrated a PASI reduction between 60 and 80% within 6 weeks. The most impressive effects were achieved with higher dosages. No rebound effect was observed after termination of the therapy. During the 6-week follow-up, only 1 patient experienced a relapse [28]. No further studies have been published so far.

Interleukin 10

IL-10 was first described in 1989 and is produced by Th2 lymphocytes, T regulatory cells, B-lymphocytes, monocytes, macrophages, eosinophils, mast cells and keratinocytes. The effects are conveyed by the IL-10 receptor. The cutaneous IL-10 mRNA expression in psoriatic lesions is significantly lower than in atopic skin or in cutaneous T cell lymphoma, but the same as in normal skin. Hence, there is a relative IL-10 deficiency in psoriatic skin [29].

The immunoregulatory function of IL-10 seems to be the limitation of inflammatory processes and a support of the humoral Th2 immune response. The APC are being blocked, as well as the production of proinflammatory mediators such as IL-1, IL-2, IL-6, TNF-α, IFN-γ, IL-8 and its receptor CXCR2. Established long-term antipsoriatic therapies, such as the use of UVB light [30] and vitamin D analogues, are able to enhance IL-10 synthesis [31]. In a phase II study, 10 patients received subcutaneous injections with recombinant human IL-10 (rhuIL-10) either at 8 μg/kg daily or 20 μg/kg 3 times a week over a period of 7 weeks with a follow-up period of 5 weeks. In 9 of 10 patients, antipsoriatic effects were observed. The efficacy was independent of the therapeitic regimen, but there was a slightly better response in the 3-times-weekly group. An average PASI reduction of 55.3% was achieved [32]. Similar results were obtained in another phase II study [33], where 10 patients were treated with 4 μg/kg rhuIL-10 daily for 6 weeks. A clinically significant improvement could be demonstrated in 9 of 10 patients. The mean PASI score reduction was 67.9% after 6 weeks. In another study, 28 patients received 20 μg/kg of rhuIL-10 s.c. 3 times a week or placebo for 12 weeks. They could confirm an efficacy after 6–8 weeks, but no sustained significant clinical improvement after 12 weeks as compared to placebo [34]. In a 4-month placebo-controlled double-blind phase-II study by Friedrich et al. [35], the long-term effect of IL-10 application was examined. Seventeen patients with plaque psoriasis in remission received either 10 μg/kg IL-10 or placebo 3 times a week until they relapsed. In the observational period, about 90% of the patients of the placebo group showed a relapse as compared to only 28.6% in the IL-10 group, indicating successful prevention of a relapse. Nevertheless, all the studies only examined a small patient cohort, and phase III studies are missing.

Interleukin-12/23 p40 Antibodies

IL-12 and IL-23 have been implicated in the pathogenesis of psoriasis. Both are heterodimeric cytokines composed of 2 subunits: IL-12 has a unique p35 subunit, IL-23 contains a p19 chain, and both share a p40 subunit. IL-12 is produced by APC like dendritic cells (DC) and activated monocytes/macrophages. It stimulates the differentiation of Th1 cells, and subsequently the secretion of IFN-γ. IL-23 skews and polarizes naïve T cells of psoriatic skin in the direction of Th17 cells, which are a distinct lineage of CD4+ effector cells [36]. The Th17 cell differentiation is initiated by transforming growth factor-β signaling in the context of IL-1β, IL-6 and TNF-α, and the survival of Th17 cells is dependent on IL-23. Th17 cells produce IL-17 and IL-22. IL-17 induces multiple proinflammatory mediators, including chemokines, cytokines and metalloproteinases from epithelial cells and fibroblasts. IL-22 increases the innate immune response, inhibits epidermal cell differentiation and, together with IL-17, enhances the expression of antimicrobial peptides [37]. One may therefore expect that an antibody against IL-12/23 p40 will affect keratinocytes as well as CD4+ T cells. Indeed, monoclonal antibodies directed against the p40 subunit shared by IL-12 and IL-23 show clinical efficacy in phase III clinical trials. In a recently published phase-III parallel double-blind placebo-controlled study, including 766 patients with moderate-to-severe psoriasis, patients were randomly assigned to receive the fully human IL-12/23 monoclonal antibody CNTO1275 (ustekinumab) 45 mg (n = 255) or 90 mg (n = 256) at weeks 0 and 4 and then every

12 weeks, or placebo (n = 255) at weeks 0 and 4, with subsequent crossover to ustekinumab at week 12. Patients who were initially randomized to receive ustekinumab at week 0 and achieved at least PASI 75 at weeks 28 and 40, were re-randomized at week 40 to maintenance ustekinumab or withdrawal from treatment until loss of response. In total, 67.1% patients in the ustekinumab 45-mg group, 66.4% receiving 90 mg ustekinumab and 3.1% receiving placebo achieved PASI 75 at week 12. At week 40, 162 patients were randomly assigned to maintenance ustekinumab, and 160 to withdrawal. PASI 75 response was better maintained (to at least 1 year) in those receiving maintenance ustekinumab than in those withdrawn from treatment at week 40. Adverse event rates were similar, the most common side effects were infections, especially of the respiratory tract [38].

In the PHOENIX2 study, which was a multicenter phase-III double-blind placebo-controlled study, 1,230 patients with moderate-to-severe psoriasis were randomly assigned to receive ustekinumab 45 mg (n = 409) or 90 mg (n = 411) at weeks 0 and 4, then every 12 weeks, or placebo (n = 410). Patients achieving ≥50 but <75% PASI improvement as compared to baseline were re-randomised at week 28 to continue dosing every 12 weeks or shorten the therapeutic interval to 8 weeks. The results showed that 66.7% of patients receiving ustekinumab 45 mg, 75.7% receiving ustekinumab 90 mg and 3.7% receiving placebo had a PASI 75 response at week 12. In the group of partial responders that were randomized to receive ustekinumab 90 mg every 8 weeks, twice as many patients achieved PASI 75 at week 52 than those who continued to receive the same dose every 12 weeks. There were no significant differences between dosing groups in the 45-mg arm. Rates of adverse events were similar in all treatment groups [39]. Ustekinumab has just received FDA and EMEA approval.

From another company, ABT-874, also an IL-12/23 p40 monoclonal antibody, is under investigation and is being tested in phase III trials at the moment. Results from a 12-week randomized double-blind placebo-controlled phase-II trial were recently published; 180 patients were included and randomized in 6 groups to receive ABT-874 or placebo as subcutaneous injections: one 200-mg dose of ABT-874 at week 0, 100 mg every other week for 12 weeks, 200 mg weekly for 4 weeks, 200 mg every other week for 12 weeks or placebo. In the group receiving 1 single injection of 200 mg ABT-874, 63% had a PASI 75 [40].

Interestingly, Lee et al. [41] examined psoriatic skin for the production of IL-23, and detected a reliable increase in p19 mRNA by quantitative reverse polymerase chain reaction in lesional as compared to nonlesional skin. The increase in p19 was 2 times higher than that observed for p40. The IL-12 subunit p35 was not elevated, indicating that: (1) antibodies directed against p40 work primarily because of their anti-IL-23 activity; (2) antibodies against p19 and/or Th17 cytokines may be equally effective, and perhaps 'safer' than an anti-p40 agent. Clinical studies will have to prove the hypothesis.

Inhibition of Proinflammatory Cytokines

Chronic inflammatory conditions often result from aberrant production of proinflammatory factors such as interleukins and chemokines. In psoriatic plaques, type 1 cytokines (such as TNF-α and IFN-γ) are present in increased concentrations; therefore, these cytokines were the first targets for therapeutic interventions. TNF-α is mainly produced by monocytes and tissue macrophages in inflammatory scenarios, as well as a lot of other cell types e.g. T and B lymphocytes, dendritic cells, keratinocytes, etc. The group of injectable TNF-α blockers (either monoclonal antibodies or receptors), such as infliximab, etanercept and adalimumab, are nowadays well established as therapies against rheumatic diseases, chronic inflammatory bowel disease as well as psoriasis. Since they will be dealt with in other chapters, we will not go into detail. There is 1 new TNF-α antibody in the pipeline, termed golimumab, which has been shown to significantly improve the signs and symptoms of psoriatic arthritis. In a randomized phase-III placebo-controlled study (n = 405), 40.4% of patients receiving 50 mg golimumab s.c. achieved a PASI 75 after 2 weeks, compared with 2.5% of patients receiving a placebo. The efficacy of the treatment lasted through week 52 and was well tolerated [42].

Other proinflammatory cytokines/chemokines that are also overexpressed in psoriasis include IL-6, IL-8 and IL-18.

Interferon-γ

IFN-γ is the only type II IFN and is upregulated in response to trauma, infection, cancer and autoimmune diseases. It is produced by Th1 lymphocytes, cytotoxic lymphocytes, natural killer cells, B cells, NKT cells and professional APC, like monocytes/macrophages and DC. The production of IFN-γ is controlled by cytokines, most notably IL-12 and IL-18. Psoriasis also shows a strong genomic signature of IFN-γ-regulated genes [43], indicating that IFN-γ blockage might be of benefit in the treatment of psoriasis. Controversial results, however, were obtained by different groups regarding serum and cutaneous levels of IFN-γ in psoriatic patients [44, 45]. The anti-IFN-γ antibody fontolizumab (HuZAF™) is currently being tested in phase II trials with patients suffering from rheumatoid arthritis. It has already been successfully used as therapy in patients with Crohn's disease [46], and could also be an attractive treatment option for psoriasis.

Interferon-α

Plasmacytoid DC (PDC), the natural IFN-α-producing cells, infiltrate the skin of psoriatic patients and become activated to produce IFN-α early during disease formation. In a xenograft model of human psoriasis, blocking IFN-α signaling or inhibiting the ability of PDC to produce IFN-α prevents the T-cell-dependent development of the disease [5]. PDC and PDC-derived IFN-α therefore represent potential targets for the treatment of psoriasis. A phase-I randomized double-blind placebo-controlled clinical trial of MEDI-545, a fully human monoclonal antibody targeting IFN-α, was conducted to examine its potential for the treatment of psoriasis, and was terminated in April 2008. Patients were dosed once intravenously (1.0, 3.0, 10.0 and 30.0 mg/kg), and subsequently evaluated for a period of 126 days, including blood and skin analysis at regular intervals. It seems to be safe, since a phase II trial is planned.

Interleukin 6

IL-6 is a multifunctional cytokine that regulates immune responses by enhancing B cell, T cell and macrophage activation, hematopoiesis, the acute phase response by stimulating the production of 'acute phase' plasma proteins by the liver, and inflammation. In addition, it is a promoter of Th17 differentiation [47]. Aberrated IL-6 production is implicated in the pathology of several disease processes, including rheumatoid arthritis (RA), systemic-onset juvenile chronic arthritis, osteoporosis and psoriasis. Increases in IL-6 mRNA and protein were observed in psoriatic plaques, and IL-6 levels were found to be elevated in the plasma of psoriasis patients. IL-6 is produced by a number of different cell types (such as dermal fibroblasts, macrophages, endothelial cells, dendritic cells and keratinocytes) in response to a variety of stimuli, which include other cytokines, such as IL-1, TNF-α and platelet-derived growth factor [48]. The humanized monoclonal anti-IL-6 antibody tocilizumab (Actemra®) has been tested in phase III clinical trials with patients suffering from RA and juvenile chronic arthritis and showed promising results. Patients treated with tocilizumab (either 4 or 8 mg/kg) plus methotrexate achieved a significant and clinically important improvement in the signs and symptoms of moderate to severe RA compared to patients treated with placebo and methotrexate [49]. No trials with psoriatic patients have been conducted up to now, but tocilizumab could also be of benefit for them.

Interleukin 8

IL-8, a member of the CXC chemokine family, is involved in chronic inflammation [50], and was initially identified as a neutrophil chemotactic and activating factor [51]. Besides being chemoattractive for granulocytes and T lymphocytes, it serves as a stimulatory factor for keratinocyte proliferation [52] and angiogenesis [53]. IL-8 can be produced by a variety of cell types involved in inflammation, including leukocytes (such as mast cells, neutrophils and T cells) as well as endothelial cells, fibroblasts and keratinocytes. Cytokines, like IL-1 and TNF-α, as well as viral and bacterial products can induce IL-8. Aberrant IL-8 production can cause chronic inflammatory conditions, as seen in RA, inflammatory bowel disease and psoriasis. Accumulation of activated neutrophils in lesional areas and elevated IL-8 production is observed in all these diseases. Due to these findings, a humanized anti-IL-8 antibody termed ABX-IL-8 was generated and tested for its antipsoriatic effects. The phase II clinical studies demonstrated a good safety profile, but only mild efficacy, which resulted in the withdrawal of ABX-IL-8 from further clinical development for this potential indication [54]. A fully human anti-IL-8 monoclonal antibody named HuMab 10F8 was examined in a single-dose escalation study followed by a 4-week multiple-dose extension in patients with palmoplantar pustulosis. The clinical disease activity, as demonstrated by a >50% reduction in the formation of fresh pustules, was significantly reduced [55]. The therapeutic potential of this antibody in diseases associated with IL-8 overexpression (e.g. psoriasis) must be further examined.

Interleukin 18

IL-18 seems to play an important role in inflammatory, infectious and autoimmune diseases. It is part of the IL-1 superfamily and is responsible for the recruitment of DC to the sites of inflammation [56]. Keratinocytes and Langerhans cells are able to produce IL-18 [57], which, together with IL-12, stimulates the release of IFN-γ in NK cells, T helper cells and cytotoxic cells [58]. Pfizer is currently testing CE-224,535, an antagonist of the P2x7 receptor, which prevents the release of IL-1 and IL-18. Only patients with RA that did not respond to methotrexate are being recruited; clinical trials with psoriatic patients are postponed at the moment.

Blocking of Leukocyte Extravasation/Trafficking

One of the early steps in the initiation and maintenance of cutaneous inflammation is the extravasation of leukocytes. It is based on the 4 steps of tethering and rolling of leukocytes, activation, adhesion/arrest and transmigration, and results from their interaction with endothelial cells via vascular adhesion molecules named selectins. Three selectins have been identified: E-, P- and L-selectin. Their expression is upregulated by proinflammatory cytokines such as IL-8, TNF-α and chemokines. Especially the interaction between E-selectin and the cutaneous lymphocyte-associated antigen on the surface of T lymphocytes plays a crucial step in 'T cell homing' to the skin. Additional adhesion is ensured by the interaction between LFA-1 on T lymphocyte surfaces and ICAM-1 on endothelial cells. Proinflammatory cytokines, such as interferon-γ and IL-1, increase ICAM-1 expression. All these steps represent important targets for therapeutic interventions. Efalizumab (Raptiva®) has already been approved as therapy for stable plaque psoriasis since 2003. It is a humanized monoclonal anti-CD11a antibody, blocking the interaction between CD11a (a subunit of LFA-1) and ICAM-1. In February 2009, after the occurrence of 3 confirmed cases of progressive multifocal leukoencephalopathy in patients treated with efalizumab, the EMEA has concluded that the benefits of efalizumab no longer outweigh its risks, and that the marketing authorization should be suspended across the European Union.

The synthetic pan-selectin antagonist bimosiamose (TBC1269) was demonstrated to be effective in preclinical models of psoriasis as well as in an open-label observational clinical pilot-trial with psoriatic patients. Five patients received subcutaneous intralesional injections of bimosiamose for 2 weeks at a daily dosage of 600 mg/day, which resulted in a reduction in epidermal thickness and lymphocyte infiltration.

The clinical improvement measured by PASI changes before and after treatment was statistically significant ($p = 0.02$) [59]. For the indications of asthma, chronic obstructive pulmonary disease and psoriasis, several phase 1 and phase 2a studies were run, treating approximately 200 volunteers and patients. In these trials, bimosiamose proved to be safe and effective. At the moment, a multicenter randomized double-blind placebo-controlled phase 2 study is being conducted testing bimosiamose 5% cream for the treatment of patients with chronic plaque type psoriasis. Another pan-selectin inhibitor named efomycine M has been developed, demonstrating reduced leukocyte adhesion in vitro and significantly diminished rolling in mouse ear venules in vivo, as seen by intravital microscopy. In addition, efomycine M alleviated cutaneous inflammation in 2 complementary mouse models of psoriasis [60]. Clinical trials are still missing.

Other Interference Strategies

Angiogenesis is a hallmark of psoriasis [61]. Dermal blood vessels in psoriatic plaques are dilated, elongated and leaky. It still remains unclear whether this type of vascular pathology is due to altered characteristics in the endothelial cells of the blood vessels themselves or is triggered by the proinflammatory environment generated by T cells. Whatever the circumstances are, proangiogenic mediators – like vascular endothelial growth factor (VEGF), hypoxia-inducible factors, TNF-α and IL-8 – are highly activated and overexpressed in psoriatic skin, and therefore attractive candidates for therapeutic intervention. The idea that antiangiogenetic strategies could be a promising approach is supported by the demonstration of antiangiogenetic activities of traditional antipsoriatic compounds, such as cyclosporine, methotrexate and vitamin D_3 analogues.

VEGF and its receptors are key players in physiological angiogenesis (e.g. embryogenesis) and in adult neovascularization. It is strongly overexpressed by keratinocytes in psoriatic skin. Furthermore, serum levels of VEGF are elevated in psoriatic patients and correlate with the degree of severity of psoriasis. Newly formed dermal blood vessels express adhesion molecules, like ICAM-1, E-selectin and vascular cell adhesion molecule 1, which enable CD4+ lymphocytes to bind and migrate into the dermis. In the skin of VEGF transgenic mice, an increased subepidermal angiogenesis with enhanced adhesion of leukocytes was observed, resulting in the development of hyperkeratotic skin lesions resembling psoriasis [62]. This phenotype was reversed by using a potent VEGF antagonist (VEGF-Trap). Two main pathways that contribute to the process of angiogenesis, i.e. matrix metalloproteases and the VEGF signaling pathway, could be blocked by AE-941 (Neovastat; Aeterna, Québec, Qué., Canada), a shark cartilage extract. In a phase-I/II single-center dose-comparison clinical trial, patients with psoriasis were randomly assigned to receive 1 of 4 doses of AE-941 (30, 60, 120 and 240 ml/day), administered orally twice daily. After the treatment duration of 12 weeks, 12.2% (6/49) had a PASI improvement of at least 30%, and 30.6% (15/49) had a PASI improvement of at least 20%. Analysis of the 30% response criteria between the low-dose (30 and 60 ml/day) and the high-dose groups (120 and 240 ml/day) showed no statistically significant difference. While further studies in psoriasis are missing, the therapeutic value of AE-941 is currently being assessed in patients with non-small-cell lung cancer.

Another attractive candidate for an antiangiogenetic intervention is TNF-α itself. Low-dose infliximab in combination with stable methotrexate therapy of psoriasis resulted in reduced VEGF expression and angiogenesis in lesional dermis, and was associated with disease improvement [63]. At the same time, infliximab significantly decreased the expression of angiopoietin, its receptor Tie-2 and matrix metalloproteinase 9, all involved in vessel growth, maturation and stabilization. It is also believed to reduce the numbers of αvβ3-positive blood vessels. Treatment with etanercept reduced VEGF serum levels of patients suffering from RA, supporting the role of TNF-α in proangiogenic processes. The development of antiangiogenic therapies that do not target the immune system would be a great advantage due to avoiding side effects of general immune suppression.

Perspectives

There is a high need for systemic antipsoriatic therapies with high and sustained efficacy, good tolerability, ease of use, cost effectiveness, long-term safety, and suitability for all ages, types of psoriasis and a widespread patient collective. None of the systemic therapies currently available fulfill all of these expectations. The better understanding of the pathogenesis causing this highly inflammatory disease opens up new perspectives for more specific therapeutic interventions. New systemic biologic approaches will allow us to assess the individual '-omic' situation in a given patient, and, as a consequence, to design novel therapies that are tailor made for each individual suffering from psoriasis.

References

1 McKenzie RC, Sabin E: Aberrant signalling and transcription factor activation as an explanation for the defective growth control and differentiation of keratinocytes in psoriasis: a hypothesis (review). Exp Dermatol 2003;12:337–345.

2 Ortonne JP: Recent developments in the understanding of the pathogenesis of psoriasis (review). Br J Dermatol 1999;140(suppl 54):1–7.

3 Zenz R, Eferl R, Kenner L, Florin L, Hummerich L, Mehic D, Scheuch H, Angel P, Tschachler E, Wagner EF: Psoriasis-like skin disease and arthritis caused by inducible epidermal deletion of Jun proteins. Nature 2005;437:369–375.

4 Prinz JC: Disease mimicry – a pathogenetic concept for T cell-mediated autoimmune disorders triggered by molecular mimicry (review)? Autoimmun Rev 2005;3:10–15.

5 Nestle FO, Conrad C, Tun-Kyi A, Homey B, Gombert M, Boyman O, Burg G, Liu Y-J, Gilliet M: Plasmacytoid predendritic cells initiate psoriasis through interferon-α production. J Exp Med 2005; 202:135–143.

6 Mommers JM, van Rossum MM, van Erp PE, van de Kerkhof PC: Changes in keratin 6 and keratin 10 (co-) expression in lesional and symptomless skin of spreading psoriasis. Dermatology 2000;201:15–20.

7 O'Neill LA: Targeting signal transduction as a strategy to treat inflammatory diseases (review). Nat Rev Drug Discov 2006;5:549–563.

8 Schneider MR, Werner S, Paus R, Wolf E: Beyond wavy hairs: the epidermal growth factor receptor and its ligands in skin biology and pathology (review). Am J Pathol 2008;173:14–24.

9 Miyagawa S, Fujimoto H, Ko S, Hirota S, Kitamura Y: Improvement of psoriasis during imatinib therapy in a patient with a metastatic gastrointestinal stromal tumour. Br J Dermatol 2002;147:406–407.

10 Robinson MJ, Cobb MH: Mitogen-activated protein kinase pathways. Curr Opin Cell Biol 1997;9:180–186.

11 Roux PP, Blenis J: ERK and p38 MAPK-activated protein kinases: a family of protein kinases with diverse biological functions (review). Microbiol Mol Biol Rev 2004;68:320–344.

12 Lee JC, Laydon JT, McDonnell PC, Gallagher TF, Kumar S, Green D, McNulty D, Blumenthal MJ, Keys JR, Land Vatter SW, Strickler JE, McLaughlin MM, Siemens IR, Fisher SM, Livi GP, White JR, Adams JL, Young PR: A protein kinase involved in the regulation of inflammatory cytokine biosynthesis. Nature 1994;372:739–746.

13 Johansen C, Kragballe K, Westergaard M, Henningsen J, Kristiansen K, Iversen L: The mitogen-activated protein kinases p38 and ERK1/2 are increased in lesional psoriatic skin. Br J Dermatol 2005;152:37–42.

14 Ding C: Drug evaluation: VX-702, a MAP kinase inhibitor for rheumatoid arthritis and acute coronary syndrome. Curr Opin Investig Drugs 2006;7: 1020–1025.

15 O'Shea JJ, Pesu M, Borie DC, Changelian PS: A new modality for immunosuppression: targeting the Jak/ Stat pathway (review). Nat Rev Drug Discov 2004;3: 555–564.

16 Sano S, Chan KS, Carbajal S, Clifford J, Peavey M, Kiguchi K, Itami S, Nickoloff BJ, DiGiovanni J: Stat3 links activated keratinocytes and immunocytes required for development of psoriasis in a novel transgenic mouse model. Nat Med 2005;11:43–49.

17 Skvara H, Dawid M, Kleyn E, Wolff B, Meingasser JG, Knight H, Dumortier T, Kopp T, Fallahi N, Stary G, Burkhart C, Grenet O, Wagner J, Hijazi Y, Morris RE, McGeown C, Rordorf C, Griffiths CE, Stingl G, Jung T: The PKC inhibitor AEB071 may be a therapeutic option for psoriasis. J Clin Invest 2008;118: 3151–3159.

18 Bos JD, Meinardi MM, van Joost T, heule F, Powles AV, Fry L: Use of cyclosporin in psoriasis (review). Lancet 1989;2:1500–1502.

19 Haider AS, Lowes MA, Suárez-Fariñas M, Zaba LC, Cardinale I, Khatcherian A, Novitskaya I, Wittkowski KM, Krueger JG: Identification of cellular pathways of 'type 1,' Th17 T cells, and TNF- and inducible nitric oxide synthase-producing dendritic cells in autoimmune inflammation through pharmacogenomic study of cyclosporine A in psoriasis. J Immunol 2008;180:1913–1920.

20 Papp K, Bissonnette R, Rosoph L, Wasel N, Lynde CW, Searles G, Shear NH, Huizinga RB, Maksymowych WP: Efficacy of ISA247 in plaque psoriasis: a randomised, multicentre, double-blind, placebo-controlled phase III study. Lancet 2008; 371:1337–1342.

21 Weinshenker BG, Bass BH, Ebers GC, Rice GP: Remission of psoriatic lesions with muromonab-CD3 (orthoclone OKT3) treatment. Am Acad Dermatol 1989;20:1132–1133.

22 Gottlieb AB, Lebwohl M, Shirin S, Sherr A, Gilleaudeau P, Singer G, Solodkina G, Grossman R, Gisoldi E, Philips S, Neisler HM, Krueger JG: Anti-CD4 monoclonal antibody treatment of moderate to severe psoriasis vulgaris: results of a pilot, multicenter, multiple-dose, placebo-controlled study. J Am Acad Dermatol 2000;43:595–604.

23 Bagel J, Garland WT, Breneman D, Holick M, Littlejohn TW, Crosby D, Faust H, Fivenson D, Nichols J: Administration of DAB389IL-2 to patients with recalcitrant psoriasis: a double-blind, phase II multicenter trial. J Am Acad Dermatol 1998;38:938–944.

24 June CH, Ledbetter JA, Linsley PS, Thompson CB: Role of the CD28 receptor in T-cell activation. Immunol Today 1990;11:211–216.

25 Abrams JR, Lebwohl MG, Guzzo CA, Jegasothy BV, Goldfarb MT, Goffe BS, Menter A, Lowe NJ, Krueger G, Brown MJ, Weiner RS, Birkhofer MJ, Warner GL, Berry KK, Linsley PS, Krueger JG, Ochs HD, Kelley SL, Khang S: CTLA4Ig-mediated blockade of T-cell costimulation in patients with psoriasis vulgaris. J Clin Invest 1999;103:1243–1252.

26 Gottlieb AB, Lebwohl M, Totoritis MC, Abdulghani AA, Shuey SR, Romano P, Chaudhari U, Allen RS, Lizambri RG: Clinical and histologic response to single-dose treatment of moderate to severe psoriasis with an anti-CD80 monoclonal antibody. J Am Acad Dermatol 2002;47:692–700.

27 Ghoreschi K, Röcken M: Immune deviation strategies in the therapy of psoriasis. Curr Drug Targets Inflamm Allergy 2004;3:193–198.

28 Ghoreschi K, Thomas P, Breit S, Dugas M, Mailhammer R, van Eden W, van der Zee R, Biedermann T, Prinz J, Mack M, Mrowietz U, Christophers E, Schlöndorff D, Plewig G, Sander CA, Röcken M: Interleukin-4 therapy of psoriasis induces Th2 responses and improves human autoimmune disease. Nat Med 2003;9:40–46.

29 Asadullah K, Sterry W, Stephanek K, Jasulaitis D, Leupold M, Audring H, Volk HD, Döcke WD: IL-10 is a key cytokine in psoriasis. Proof of principle by IL-10 therapy: a new therapeutic approach. J Clin Invest 1998;101:783–794.

30 Shreedhar V, Giese T, Sung VW, Ullrich SE: A cytokine cascade including prostaglandin E2, IL-4, and IL-10 is responsible for UV-induced systemic immune suppression. J Immunol 1998;160:3783–3789.

31 Michel G, Gailis A, Jarzebska-Deussen B, Müschen A, Mirmohammadsadegh A, Ruzicka T: 1,25-(OH)2-vitamin D_3 and calcipotriol induce IL-10 receptor gene expression in human epidermal cells. Inflamm Res 1997;46:32–34.

32 Asadullah K, Döcke WD, Ebeling M, Friedrich M, Belbe G, Audring H, Volk HD, Sterry W: Interleukin 10 treatment of psoriasis: clinical results of a phase 2 trial. Arch Dermatol 1999;135:187–192.

33 Reich K, Brück M, Gräfe A, Vente C, Neumann C, Garbe C: Treatment of psoriasis with interleukin-10. J Invest Dermatol 1998;111:1235–1236.

34 Kimball AB, Kawamura T, Tejura K, Boss C, Hancox AR, Vogel JC, Steinberg SM, Turner ML, Blauvelt A: Clinical and immunologic assessment of patients with psoriasis in a randomized, double-blind, placebo-controlled trial using recombinant human interleukin 10. Arch Dermatol 2002;138:1341–1346.

35 Friedrich M, Döcke WD, Klein A, Philipp S, Volk HD, Sterry W, Asadullah K: Immunomodulation by interleukin-10 therapy decreases the incidence of relapse and prolongs the relapse-free interval in psoriasis. J Invest Dermatol 2002;118:672–677.

36 Park H, Li Z, Yang XO, Chang SH, Nurieva R, Wang Y-H, Wang Y, Hood L, Zhu Z, Tian Q, Dong C: A distinct lineage of CD4 T cells regulates tissue inflammation by producing interleukin 17. Nat Immunol 2005;6:1133–1141.

37 McKenzie BS, Kastelein RA, Cua DJ: Understanding the IL-23-IL-17 immune pathway. Trends Immunol 2006;27:17–23.

38 Leonardi CL, Kimball AB, Papp KA, Yeilding N, Guzzo C, Wang Y, Li S, Dooley LT, Gordon KB, PHOENIX 1 study investigators: Efficacy and safety of ustekinumab, a human interleukin-12/23 monoclonal antibody, in patients with psoriasis: 76-week results from a randomised, double-blind, placebo-controlled trial (PHOENIX 1). Lancet 2008;371: 1665–1674.

39 Papp KA, Langley RG, Lebwohl M, Krueger GG, Szapary P, Yeilding N, Guzzo C, Hsu MC, Wang Y, Li S, Dooley LT, Reich K, PHOENIX 2 study investigators: Efficacy and safety of ustekinumab, a human interleukin-12/23 monoclonal antibody, in patients with psoriasis: 52-week results from a randomised, double-blind, placebo-controlled trial (PHOENIX 2). Lancet 2008;371:1675–1684.

40 Kimball AB, Gordon KB, Langley RG, Menter A, Chartash EK, Valdes J, ABT-874 Psoriasis Study Investigators: Safety and efficacy of ABT-874, a fully human interleukin 12/23 monoclonal antibody, in the treatment of moderate to severe chronic plaque psoriasis: results of a randomized, placebo-controlled, phase 2 trial. Arch Dermatol 2008;144:200–207.

41 Lee E, Trepicchio WL, Osterreicher JL, Pittman D, Wang F, Chamian F, Dhodapkar M, Krueger JG: Increased expression of interleukin 23 p19 and p40 in lesional skin of patients with psoriasis vulgaris. J Exp Med 2004;199:125–130.

42 Kavanaugh A, McInnes I ,Mease P: Golimumab, a new human TNF-alpha antibody administered as a monthly subcutaneous injection in psoriatic arthritis: 24 week efficacy and safety results of the randomized, placebo controlled GO-REVEAL study. Abstract 62nd Eur League Rheum, Paris, 2008.

43 Lew W, Bowcock AM, Krueger JG: Psoriasis vulgaris: cutaneous lymphoid tissue supports T-cell activation and 'type 1' inflammatory gene expression. Trends Immunol 2004;25:295–305.

44 Gomi T, Shiohara T, Munataka T, Imanishi K, Nagashima M: IL-1α, TNF- α and IFN-γ in psoriasis. Arch Dermatol 1991;127:827–830.

45 Uyemura K, Yamamura M, Fivenson DF, Modlin RL, Nickoloff BJ: The cytokine network in lesional and lesion-free psoriatic skin is characterized by a T-helper type-1 cell-mediated response. J Invest Dermatol 1993;101:701–705.

46 Hommes DW, Mikhajlova TL, Stoinov S, Stimac D, Vucelic B, Lonovics J, Zákuciová M, D'Haens G, Van Assche G, Ba S, Lee S, Pearce T: Fontolizumab, a humanised anti-interferon-gamma antibody, demonstrates safety and potential clinical activity in patients with moderate to severe Crohn's disease. Gut 2006;55:1131–1137.

47 Bettelli E, Carrier Y, Gao W, Korn T, Strom TB, Oukka M, Weiner HL, Kuchroo VK: Reciprocal developmental pathways for the generation of pathogenic effector TH17 and regulatory T cells. Nature 2006;441:235–238.

48 Grossman RM, Krueger J, Yourish D, Granelli-Piperno A, Murphy DP, May LT, Kupper TS, Sehgal PB, Gottlieb AB: Interleukin 6 is expressed in high levels in psoriatic skin and stimulates proliferation of cultured human keratinocytes. Proc Natl Acad Sci USA 1989;86:6367–6371.

49 Maini RN, Taylor PC, Szechinski J, Pavelka K, Bröll J, Balint G, Emery P, Raemen F, Petersen J, Smolen J, Thomson D, Kishimoto T: Double-blind randomized controlled clinical trial of the interleukin-6 receptor antagonist, tocilizumab, in European patients with rheumatoid arthritis who had an incomplete response to methotrexate. Arthritis Rheum 2006;54:2817–2829.

50 Harada A, Mukaida N, Matsushima K: Interleukin 8 as a novel target for intervention therapy in acute inflammatory diseases. Mol Med Today 1996;2:482–489.

51 Yoshimura T, Matsushima K, Tanaka S, Robinson EA, Appella E, Oppenheim JJ, Leonard EJ: Purification of a human monocyte-derived neutrophil chemotactic factor that has peptide sequence similarity to other host defense cytokines. Proc Natl Acad Sci USA 1987;84:9233–9237.

52 Tuschil A, Lam C, Haslberger A, Lindley I: Interleukin-8 stimulates calcium transients and promotes epidermal cell proliferation. J Invest Dermatol 1992;99:294–298.

53 Koch AE, Polverini PJ, Kunkel SL, Harlow LA, DiPietro LA, Elner VM, Elner SG, Strieter RM: Interleukin-8 as a macrophage-derived mediator of angiogenesis. Science 1992;258:1798–1801.

54 Homey B: Chemokines and chemokine receptors as targets in the therapy of psoriasis. Curr Drug Targets Inflamm Allergy 2004;3:169–174.

55 Skov L, Beurskens FJ, Zachariae C, Reitamo S, Teeling J, Satijn D, Knudsen KM, Boot E, Hudson D, Baadsgaard O, Parren P, van de Winkel: IL-8 as antibody therapeutic target in inflammatory diseases: reduction of clinical activity in palmoplantar pustulosis. J Immunol 2008;181:669–679.

56 Gutzmer R, Langer K, Mommert S, Wittmann M, Kapp A, Werfel T: Human dendritic cells express the IL-18R and are chemoattracted to IL-18. J Immunol 2003;171:6363–6371.

57 Naik SM, Cannon G, Burbach GJ, Singh SR, Swerlick RA, Wilcox JN, Ansel JC, Caughman SW: Human keratinocytes constitutively express interleukin-18 and secrete biologically active interleukin-18 after treatment with pro-inflammatory mediators and dinitrochlorobenzene. J Invest Dermatol 1999;113: 766–772.

58 Nakahira M, Ahn HJ, Park WR, Gao P, Tomura M, Park CS, Hamaoka T, Ohta T, Kurimoto M, Fujiwara H: Synergy of IL-12 and IL-18 for IFN-gamma gene expression: IL-12-induced STAT4 contributes to IFN-gamma promoter activation by up-regulating the binding activity of IL-18-induced activator protein 1. J Immunol 2002;168:1146–1153.

59 Friedrich M, Bock D, Philipp S, Ludwig N, Sabat R, Wolk K, Schroeter-Maas S, Aydt E, Kang S, Dam TN, Zahlten R, Sterry W, Wolff G: Pan-selectin antagonism improves psoriasis manifestation in mice and man. Arch Dermatol Res 2006;297:345–351.

60 Schön MP, Krahn T, Schön M, Rodriguez ML, Antonicek H, Schultz JE, Ludwig RJ, Zollner TM, Bischoff E, Bremm KD, Schramm M, Henninger K, Kaufmann R, Gollnick HP, Parker CM, Boehncke WH: Efomycine M, a new specific inhibitor of selectin, impairs leukocyte adhesion and alleviates cutaneous inflammation. Nat Med 2002;8:366–372.

61 Heidenreich R, Röcken M, Ghoreschi K: Angiogenesis: the new potential target for the therapy of psoriasis? Drug News Perspect 2008;21:97–105.

62 Detmar M, Brown LF, Schön MP, Elicker BM, Velasco P, Richard L, Fukumura D, Monsky W, Claffey KP, Jain RK: Increased microvascular density and enhanced leukocyte rolling and adhesion in the skin of VEGF transgenic mice. J Invest Dermatol 1998;111:1–6.

63 Goedkoop AY, Kraan MC, Picavet DI, de Rie MA, Teunissen MB, Bos JD, Tak PP: Deactivation of endothelium and reduction in angiogenesis in psoriatic skin and synovium by low dose infliximab therapy in combination with stable methotrexate therapy: a prospective single-centre study. Arthritis Res Ther 2004;6:R326–R334.

Georg Stingl, MD
Division of Immunology, Allergy and Infectious Diseases, Department of Dermatology, Medical University of Vienna
Währinger Gürtel 18–20
AT–1090 Vienna (Austria)
Tel. +43 1 4040 07704, Fax +43 1 4040 07574, E-Mail georg.stingl@meduniwien.ac.at

Author Index

Subject Index